EYE MOVEMENTS AND THE FUNDAMENTAL READING PROCESS

ABOUT THE AUTHOR

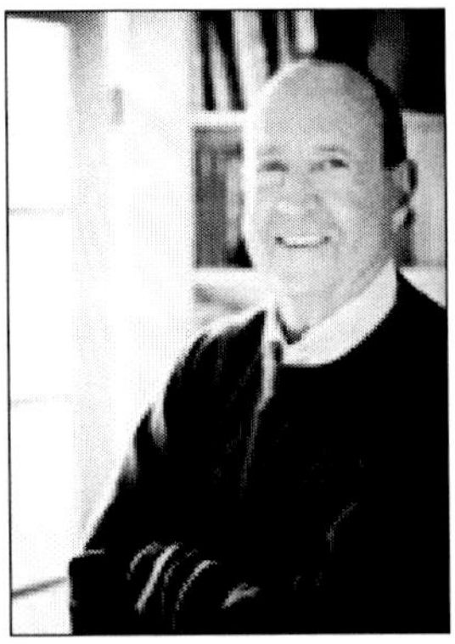

Stanford E. Taylor, M. A.

Founder, Chairman

Reading Plus/Taylor Associates/ Communications, Inc.

Stanford E. Taylor is the founder of Taylor Associates and principal designer of the Reading Plus system. Prior to establishing Taylor Associates, Mr. Taylor was founder and president of Educational Development Laboratories, Inc. (EDL/McGraw-Hill) and subsequently Instructional/Communications Technology, Inc.

A pioneer in the introduction and use of technology to improve reading/listening in the classroom, Mr. Taylor designed, manufactured, and distributed a variety of reading improvement devices; initiated the concept of the reading lab; and introduced the first mobile reading lab.

He previously served as a reading technology supervisor in the Bethpage, New York, schools, a reading technology instructor at Wagner College in Staten Island, New York, director of the Amackassin School in Blairstown, New Jersey, director of the Taylor Center for Reading Research in Huntington, New York, and comprehension skills editor for *Popular Science* magazine. He is an honorary member of the International Reading Association and the author of the National Education Association publication, "What Research Says to the Classroom Teacher about Listening." Mr. Taylor has published numerous articles for American Education Research Association journals and contributed to the publication of over 300 books and instructional programs in the area of reading.

EYE MOVEMENTS AND THE FUNDAMENTAL READING PROCESS

How to Evaluate Silent Reading Efficiency

By

STANFORD E. TAYLOR, M.A.

Taylor Associates/Communications

CHARLES C THOMAS • PUBLISHER, LTD.
Springfield • Illinois • U.S.A.

Published and Distributed Throughout the World by

CHARLES C THOMAS • PUBLISHER, LTD.
2600 South First Street
Springfield, Illinois 62704

ISBN 978-0-398-08753-1 (paper)
ISBN 978-0-398-08754-8 (ebook)

Library of Congress Catalog Card Number: 2013014842

With THOMAS BOOKS *careful attention is given to all details of manufacturing and design. It is the Publisher's desire to present books that are satisfactory as to their physical qualities and artistic possibilities and appropriate for their particular use.* THOMAS BOOKS *will be true to those laws of quality that assure a good name and good will.*

Printed in the United States of America
CR-R-3

Library of Congress Cataloging-in-Publication Data

Taylor, Stanford E. (Stanford Earl), 1927-
Eye movements and the fundamental process : how to evaluate silent reading efficiency / by Stanford E. Taylor, M.A.
pages cm
Includes bibliographical references and index.
ISBN 978-0-08753-1 (pbk.) -- ISBN 978-0-398-08754-8 (ebook) 1. Silent reading. 2. Eye--Movements. I. Title.

LB1050.55T394 2013
372.45'4--dc23

2013014842

This book is dedicated to the memory of my father, Earl A. Taylor, whose pioneering work in the area of eye-movement recording and explanation of the Fundamental Reading Process skills inspired my work over the years in these areas and to my son, Stanford Mark Taylor, who continues the legacy in reading technology to develop fluency in silent reading

FOREWORD

Stanford Taylor is one of our nation's leading experts on the role of the eye in reading and the technologies that are available to record and evaluate eye movements during reading. He is correct in his observation that there is a general lack of knowledge about the Fundamental Reading Process and how eye movements influence the efficiency of silent reading. This book will help to overcome this knowledge deficiency by providing essential information to those in higher education who prepare students for the teaching profession, to teachers in the classroom who help students learn to read, to reading clinics, and to behavioral optometrists who work with students who are experiencing unusual visual problems during reading. Within the pages of this book one can find information on such topics as the Fundamental Reading Process, the history of eye-movement recording, and how to interpret the data that can be derived from eye-movement devices such as the Visagraph.

Stanford Taylor's credentials testify as to why he is considered to be a leading scholar in the field of reading for more than half a century. He has been the founder of several organizations that developed cutting-edge reading instructional programs, and these organizations brought these programs to thousands of schools where they are used to introduce students to reading and to help them become more highly skilled readers. To add to Stanford Taylor's versatility as a creative scholar he has also invented and developed instruments to record the movements of the eye while reading and has had patents awarded for these inventions. To add to his accomplishments, he has a wide list of publications that explain how the eye functions during silent reading.

Stan and I have collaborated on many papers and projects in the past to call attention to the need for more awareness about the nature of fluency in silent reading and the role that automaticity in word recognition plays as a prerequisite for fluency. This book will add to this information base.

In summary, this book by Stanford Taylor is essential reading for all who want to understand the role of the eye in silent reading and want to increase their instructional capability as teachers and reading remediation specialists.

S. Jay Samuels, Ed.D.
Professor
Department of Educational Psychology and Curriculum and Instruction
University of Minnesota

PREFACE

There has long been an absence in the annals of reading development in terms of the most basic reading skills, which this author terms the Fundamental Reading Process, as well as a lack of appreciation of what can be easily measured through eye-movement recording during silent reading.

With the relative ease of use of today's eye-movement recording techniques and the core curriculum's demand for explicit and accurate measurements of the reading process, it is essential that eye-movement recording be utilized by all schools as a quick and easy means of selecting students who need silent reading fluency development. In addition these same recordings can indicate the need for possible referrals to a vision specialist when visual/functional impediments are extreme.

The purpose of this book is multi-faceted; it is primarily dedicated to exploring the nature of the Fundamental Reading Process and to discussing the manner in which proficiency in these basic skills can be evaluated through eye-movement recording. Here is a brief overview of the contents of this book:

- Understanding the nature of the Fundamental Reading Process
- History of eye-movement recording
- Exploring eye-movement recording through the use of the Visagraph Eye-Movement Recording system
  - Selecting the reading test level
  - Interpreting the Reading Report
    - Fixations
    - Regressions
    - Average span of recognition
    - Average duration of fixation
    - Reading rate
    - Grade level efficiency
    - Cross-correlation
  - Reading simulation
  - Graphs

    - Interpreting the Visual/Functional Report
- Uses of eye movements in terms of reading appraisal
- Field use of the Visagraph Eye Movement Recording system (schools, clinics, optometrists)
- Visagraph/EyeLink comparison in terms of eye-movement data
- 2012 Visagraph Norm Study Report

Reading and tutoring centers will naturally be interested in both the diagnostic eye-movement recording techniques as well as the web-based practice techniques available through computer technology. The ability for clients to use this silent reading development technology at home, beyond usual clinic hours, is certainly an advantage in terms of reading remediation.

Reading researchers might also be intrigued by the comprehensive description of the silent reading process, as well as the effect on the oral reading process with the development of proficiency in silent reading. Especially helpful should be the information revealed through eye-movement recordings about the many subliminal factors involved in the process of reading, as well as the changes produced by today's web-based computer techniques to modify the basic visual/functional, perceptual, and information-processing skills that comprise the silent reading process.

In addition higher education curriculum directors may be interested in this book as recommended reading for graduate courses that cover what occurs during silent reading and what outcomes are possible with current reading practice programs using web-based computer technology. Such programs might also be of interest for their use with incoming freshmen who need to improve their silent reading proficiency to deal with the more extensive and higher-level content they will encounter in their post-secondary education.

Classroom teachers may be particularly interested in the chapters that describe what has and can be been done in classrooms and labs to improve silent reading proficiency.

ACKNOWLEDGMENTS

My sincere thanks to the educators, clinicians, and vision specialists who were able to provide very detailed information on their use of the Visagraph for inclusion in this book. I wish to thank them also for the value they place on the Visagraph as an important tool that assists them in their profession.

Thank you to Maret Felzien, MA, Reading Specialist/Associate Professor at Northeastern Junior College; to Sheri Kennedy, School Psychological Examiner Poplar Bluff Kindergarten Center (PBKC) in Poplar Bluff, Missouri; and to Holly Voorhees Carmical who is the Curriculum Coordinator for Douglas County, Colorado. My appreciation is extended to Stacy Dean, President of Dean's Learning Center, Hamilton, New Jersey; to Tom Kroeger, Optimum Reading, LLC, Livonia, Michigan; to Megan Hudson D.C., Center Director, Brain Balance Achievement Center of West Springfield, West Springfield, Massachusetts; to Mira Halpert, M.Ed., 3D Learner Inc., Boca Raton, Florida; and to Pat Rosenbury, Brainlinking, Inc., Sandy, Utah. Finally, I wish to thank Leonard J. Press, OD, FCOVD, FAAO, Optometric Director, The Vision & Learning Center, Fair Lawn, New Jersey; to Doug Major, OD, FCOVD, El Paso de Robles School, Paso Robles, California; to Barry Tannen, OD, FCOVD, FAAO, EyeCare Professionals, PC, Hamilton Square, New Jersey; to Charles E. Shearer, OD, Bernell Corporation, Mishawaka, Indiana; to Darrell G. Schlange, OD, DOS, FAAO, Associate Professor of Optometry, Pediatrics/Binocular Vision, Illinois College of Optometry, Illinois Eye Institute Chicago, Illinois; to Joseph Sullivan, OD, FCOVD, Wichita, Kansas; to John A. Thomas, MS, OD, FCOVD, DP, Neuro-Optometric Rehabilitation, Diplomate, American Board of Disability Analysts, Professor, Adjunct, Pacific University College of Optometry, Wheat Ridge, Colorado; to Lynn F. Hellerstein, OD, FAAO, FCOVD, Hellerstein and Brenner Vision Center, PC, Centennial, Colorado; to Alan P Pearson OD, Med, PhD, FCOVD, Vision Clinics of Development and Learning, Bothell, Washington; and to Theodore S. Kadet, OD, FCOVD, Developmental Vision Associates, PLLC/dba Hope Clinic, Bellevue, Washington.

CONTENTS

EYE MOVEMENTS AND THE FUNDAMENTAL READING PROCESS

Chapter 1

EYE MOVEMENTS AND THE FUNDAMENTAL READING PROCESS

The Fundamental Reading Process is comprised of the most basic functions of reading, silent or oral. The purpose of this chapter is to acquaint the reader with these skill areas.

First, there is a reader's visual/functional capability in terms of visual acuity (ability to see clearly), binocular coordination (ability to use both eyes as a team), oculomotility (ability to easily rotate the eyes and not the head), and accuracy in tracking (directional attack employed during reading). These factors affect the clarity of print, ease, and comfort in reading, the ability to stay on lines of print, and the ability to move accurately and sequentially across each line of words during reading. These visual abilities impact the accuracy in which words are perceived and also affect feelings of ease and comfort during reading.

Reinforcement for the need for well-developed visual/functional skills is found in many references.

According to Taylor (1966):

> Reading requires that the individual give attention to the task with his whole mind and body, while, at the same time, he uses in concert a number of acquired mechanical and interpretive skills. . . .
>
> Reading efficiency is not only dependent upon the ability to see and interpret printed materials, but also upon the ability of the individual to use his two eyes together effectively, make the necessary rapid ocular rotations, and sustain effort during extended periods of near-point application. . . .

According to Taylor and Solan (1956):

> Teachers can do a great deal in the classroom to develop and improve the reading and visual efficiency of the pupils. . . . Visual experiences can be made more meaningful with careful guidance. Most individuals can be trained to see more easily, more rapidly, more accurately, and more objectively.

According to Gates (1935):

> In reading, however, a definite direction must be habituated to permit accurate perception. That the direction must be from left to right across the line has been recognized. This rule is rather unique in visual perception during reading. That pupils need to be taught and guided in forming the habit of moving the eyes consistently along the line from left to right is now obvious. Children who do not learn to do this in the initial stages of reading are certain to encounter serious difficulty in learning to read. . . . Actually the consistent left-to-right procedure is very unnatural in the sense that it has been rarely, if ever, required in any other perceptual activities engaged in by the child. Hence, the need for careful guidance.

According to Betts (1946):

> Reading cannot be brought to full fruition as a learning aid until the mechanics have been controlled. . . . Such mechanics as left-to-right progression, accurate return sweeps, and accurate word recognition skills are fundamental to reading, but they must become automatic.

Storm and Smith (1930) reported that:

> . . . the task of the school is plainly that of converting the raw material of the child's short, irregular, regressive movements and long pauses into the refined habits of the good mature reader which are characterized by the eye moving across the page in a series of broad rhythmical movements, pausing for a fraction of a second at regular points along the line to gather up as many words as possible at a glance, proceeding on to the end of the line with no regressive movements, and returning to the beginning of the next line with an accurate return sweep.

Symptoms of a lack of visual/functional competence include the following:

- Bringing the book very close to the eyes during reading
- Tilting the head to favor one eye
- Reporting visual discomfort
- Experiencing headaches from reading
- Losing one's place within the lines of print
- Moving the head instead of moving the eyes in reading
- Being easily distracted

These symptoms are cited by Maples and Hoenes (2009), as related to the College of Vision Development Quality of Life Checklist.

The near point activity of reading is not a natural human act. Humans are basically designed for distance viewing. Unfortunately, most people do not possess the visual competence required for efficient reading. Present estimates are that 30 to 60 percent of students and adults suffer, in varying degrees, from a lack of adequate visual coordination skills, poor ocular motility, and inaccurate visual tracking. The National PTA's (1999) resolution, *Learning Related Vision Problems*, states, "Knowledge regarding the relationship between poorly developed visual skills and poor academic performance is not widely held among students, parents, teachers, administrators, and public health officials." Those students classified as underachievers suffer more dramatically from a lack of such visual competence and would benefit from visual retraining. In-school visual training programs such as those administered by Hellerstein, Danner, Maples, Press, Schneebeck, and Miller (2001) and Hoover and Harris (1997) also document the value of visual training combined with computerized reading fluency development training, and both involve the use of eye-movement recording in pre- and post-testing.

Computerized visual skills practice that employs timed scanning of numbers, letters, and words followed by left-to-right displays of reading selections can improve visual/functional competence resulting in greater ease and comfort in reading, as well as more sequential input of words into short-term memory. An eye-movement study by Schlange, Patel, and Caden (1999), in which computerized fluency training that provided timed and directed left-to-right presentations of print without the support of specific visual/functional training also developed higher levels of visual/functional efficiency as revealed by pre- and post-measurements of eye-movement behavior.

Next, the aspect of perceptual efficiency, or the ability of a reader to quickly and accurately realize the orthography (letters, letter order, and letter cluster awareness) of words, the degree of automaticity of word recognition, and the ability to retain word images for a reasonable length of time during the realization of syntax directly affects comprehension and rate of reading.

According to LaBerge and Samuels (1973), Logan (1997), and Samuels (2006), if most of the time and mental effort during a fixation are required to decode or recognize a word, or if a student devotes several fixations to recognizing a word, little time or capacity is left for comprehension.

Support for responses to letters and words so that attention during reading can be directed to deriving meaning can be found in many references.

Huey (1908) reported:

> To perceive an entire new word or other combination of strokes requires considerable time, close attention, and is likely to be imperfectly done. . . . [Practice, however,] progressively frees the mind from attention to details, and makes facile the total act, shortens the time, and reduces the extent to which consciousness must concern itself with the process.

According to James (1890):

> How many ideas or things can be attended to at once. . . . Not easily more than one, unless the processes are very habitual. . . . Where, however, the processes are less automatic . . . there must be a rapid oscillation of the mind from one to the next, and no consequent gain in time.
>
> . . . we are able to process only one thing at a time, except when the processes involved have been so well learned that they can be carried out automatically.

According to Norman and Bobrow (1975):

> A considerable amount of conscious effort is often required to perform an unfamiliar task. However, when the task is repeatedly practiced, per-

> formance becomes increasingly automatic, and less conscious effort is required. Thus practice can result in increased processing efficiency, that is, increased performance with no extra allocation of resources.

Further, West (1978) stated:

> As proficiency in reading is acquired, the numerous component processes involved in reading become increasingly efficient in their use of limited attentional resources. Thus skilled readers need to allocate only a minimal amount of attentional resources to lower-level processes as they read. As a result, their comprehension is normally high, because their attentional resources can be directed almost entirely to the meaning of written passages. . . . In contrast, beginning readers must allocate a considerably larger amount of their attentional resources to lower-level processes. Indeed, for beginning readers, the portion of their attentional resources consumed by lower-level activities may be so large that they often pay insufficient attention to the meanings of written passages. As a result, their reading is likely to be awkward and slow, and their comprehension is likely to be low.

As one reads, there is an awareness of a flow of words and ideas, but the reader is unaware that this flow of information is created through a series of extremely brief visual impressions received each time the eyes pause during reading. Without conscious direction, the eyes shift position across each line of print, pausing three to five times per second to accomplish word perceptions.

The reader experiences what seems to be a continuous flow of words, in part because these visual impressions overlap each other so rapidly that they create the impression of an uninterrupted flow of text. Further, eye movements and pauses are not detected because vision drops dramatically just prior to the movement of the eyes and quickly recovers when the eyes become stationary again, as cited by Gross, Vaughan, and Valenstein (1967). This prevents the reader from sensing the blur that typically occurs during eye movements that might suggest separate impressions.

Although we read through a series of small glimpses of print, no one is aware of any real limitations as to the number of words seen at any one time. Many people mistakenly feel that they can see phrases (or even complete lines of print) at a single glance. However, from each eye pause, vision and perceptual limitations dramatically restrict what can be seen and saved to a typical average of just a single word, and with beginning readers, less than a word, as cited by Taylor, Frackenpohl, and Pettee (1960).

While reading, you may be aware of rereading content that was not understood, but seldom, if ever, are you aware of regressions (reverse eye movements). Most readers employ a multitude of split-second right-to-left eye movements that are immediately followed by recovery left-to-right eye movements as shown in the following illustration.

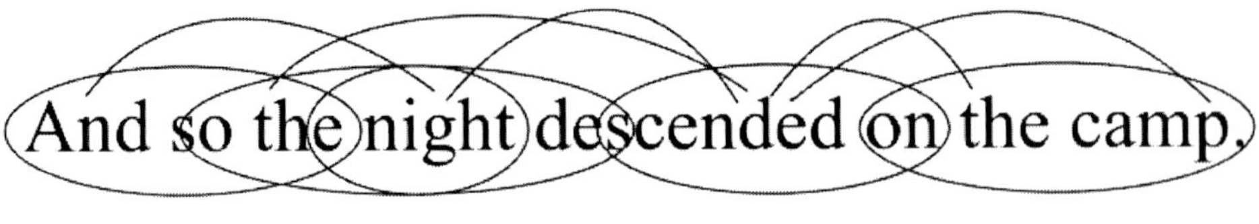

Figure 1.1

According to Taylor et al. (1960), these regressions and their recovery return movements can consume one-third or more of total reading time and up to one-half of a beginning reader's total reading time. Regressions do not aid understanding. Rather, they inhibit and confuse perception of what is read and steal time and cognitive resources in the process. The nature of the oculomotor activity employed when reading, the number of eye pauses per word, the degree of habitual regression, and even the average length of eye-pause time are behaviors acquired by trial and error during the years when one learns to read. In addition, a lack of perceptual efficiency will also affect spelling, as well as fluency, in silent reading.

Symptoms of poor perceptual efficiency in reading include the following:

- Difficulty in recognizing the orthography of words
- Poor visual memory
- Slow and labored decoding of words
- Confusing words with other words

Computerized training practice that involves the flashing (tachistoscopic exposures) of groups of letters, numbers, and core vocabulary words can improve orthographic awareness, increase automaticity of word recognition, and develop an improved visual memory, all leading to a greater amount of time during each fixation to devote to understanding and comprehension. Aiken (1896), Cattell (1885), and Volkmann (1859), and later Davis (1956), Rusk (1915), Weber (1937), and Wilkins (1917) all documented the value of tachistoscopic practice on word recognition, reading, and learning.

Lastly, the aspect of information processing effectiveness, which encompasses the manner in which words are input into short-term memory in terms of rate and sequence, directly affects the reader's ability to realize proper phrasing and syntax during reading.

Information processing relates to a student's "graduation" from word-by-word reading to a rapid awareness of word clusters as phrases and other intra-sentence structures. Reinforcement for the need to attain these skills is found in the following references:

California State Department of Education's *Handbook for Planning an Effective Reading Program* (1979) states:

> Since meaningful language occurs in units, such as phrases, sentences, and paragraphs, readers must be able to process these units of language in a rhythm similar to that used in oral communication. That is, reading must "flow" just as talking flows.

Chomsky (1976) further states:

> What they [the students] need is to shift their focus from the individual word to connected discourse and to integrate their fragmented knowledge. It is the larger picture that they need help with, in learning to attend to the semantics and syntax of a written passage, and in developing reliance on using contextual clues from the sentence or even longer passages as they read.

The series of word impressions received during every second of reading are processed through short-term memory at the reader's reading rate and in the order in which they are perceived. These word impressions are either realized as properly sequenced expressions of language or they are resequenced (not consciously) if they are received out of order as a result of regressions. Individual words must be quickly chunked (associated) into larger units of language in order for them to be finally realized mentally as phrases, complete sentences, and eventually as larger messages. If understanding is not achieved, there will be a conscious need to reread to clarify meaning.

The function of short-term memory is to deliver an accurate literal message to the mind. However, this is not a process that can be controlled and/or directed. The reader can be aware only of the outcome of this process.

There are limitations to the capability of short-term memory that affect retention and literal understanding. Typically short-term memory can hold only a maximum of five to seven items (perhaps partial impressions of words) at any one time and only for intervals of three to four seconds, as cited by Miller (1956). Beyond these limits, loss of items occurs. These limitations make it vital that the reader be able to recognize words rapidly and accurately, in proper sequence, and then quickly chunk words into larger syntactical units to minimize the number of items in short-term memory so retention can be maintained and understanding can be comprehensive.

Average adult readers, reading at approximately 250 words per minute, input four or more word impressions per second into short-term memory. They chunk words fairly rapidly (phrasing) and realize sentences ranging from 12 to 24 words in four to eight seconds. If some words are lost in this process, these readers will compensate by using their greater capability with context to complete meaning with relative accuracy. By contrast, a very accomplished reader (450 to 500 words per minute) will realize the same sentences in just two to three seconds. However, a beginning reader may require 15 seconds or more to process a 12-word sentence. Beginning or struggling readers will also lose many word impressions as they pass through short-term memory because they do not possess the contextual capability to salvage meaning as well as a more advanced reader.

A logical question is whether a reader really does need to see all the words to read. For complete accuracy in reading, the answer to this question must be yes. The fact that all words must be seen does not mean that the same attention will be devoted to each and every word. However, recognition of the meaning and significance of individual words (and later chunked words and phrases) occurs many seconds after the words have been perceived and are being processed through short-term memory. Long-term memory (experiential background) will then finally interpret the meaning, significance, and importance of the words read and the literal messages derived.

Some symptoms of poor information processing include the following:

- Slow reading rate
- Problems in reading words sequentially
- Difficulty in realizing phrases in reading
- Poor comprehension

There is no more accurate means of evaluating a reader's silent reading efficiency or fluency than through eye-movement recording, as shown in the following image of the Visagraph eye-movement recording device. Timed reading can measure rate, but not the visual and perceptual processes that result in the reading rate. Further, most standardized and state reading tests simply measure the outcome of reading and thus only reflect effectiveness, not the process of reading.

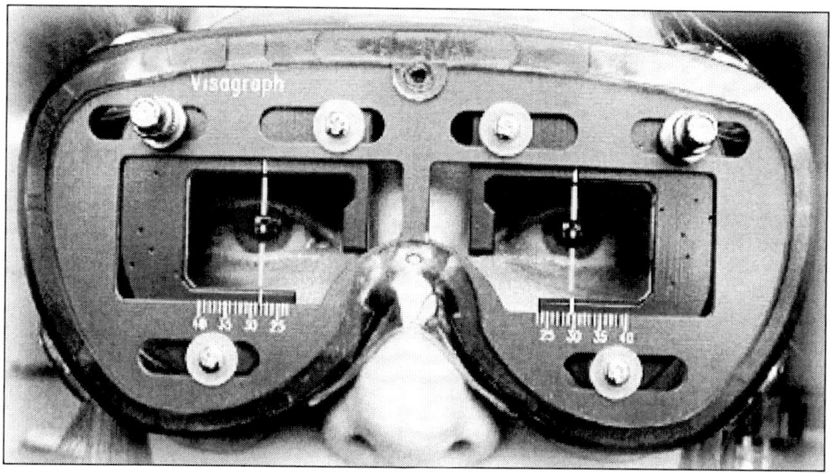

Figure 1.2

This book has been written to create an awareness of the Fundamental Reading Process (FRP) skills that a reader employs, largely in a subliminal manner, in reading any form of content, and to show how these FRP skills can be easily analyzed through eye-movement recording.

A student's oculomotor activity, as displayed through eye-movement recording, reflects the level of competency of a student's FRP. The number of fixations (eye pauses), regressions (reverse fixations), and average duration of fixation reflect a student's perceptual accuracy and efficiency and perhaps a deficit in binocular coordination. A poor reading rate, repeat reading, and a poor directional attack reflect inadequate information processing, which directly impinges on literal comprehension and ultimately higher-level cognitive processes.

Unlike oral reading fluency assessments, such as the DIBELS test, which analyzes word recognition accuracy, rate of reading, and prosody, eye-movement recordings can evaluate specific data that show exactly what the eyes do during silent reading. Such assessments reflect the visual/functional and perceptual efficiency of the reader's performance, which is key to understanding the manner in which print is perceived and the ultimate affect on comprehension.

Reading is a highly complex process, involving close interaction among the visual/functional, perceptual, and cognitive functions. A reader's eyes coordinate as they move along the lines of print in a left-to-right fashion, pausing three to five times per second to perceive words or word parts that are continuously added up into thought units, such as phrases or larger syntactical units. The reader then interprets what is read in light of his or her experiential background, associates information, and projects beyond it in terms of association, evaluations, judgments, applications, and conclusions.

Through the recording and analysis of a student's eye movements, or oculomotor activity, a reading teacher or a reading diagnostician can make objective and accurate evaluations concerning a reader's efficiency and indirect judgment about his or her effectiveness. This information can be used in prescribing a program of silent reading fluency development to remedy or correct deficiencies in visual functioning, perception, and cognition. As reading improves during fluency development training, eye-movement recording can also be used, in conjunction with teacher evaluations and standardized tests, to measure changes to document the efficiency and effectiveness of the total reading process.

Key points to note regarding eye movements are:

- Reflections of reading efficiency
- Predictions about reading effectiveness
- Reflections of visual/functional, perceptual, and cognitive adaptations over time
- Ease and comfort during reading and the ability to sustain attention

CONCLUSION

The visual/functional, perceptual, and information processing skills a reader employs during each second of reading will largely determine the degree to which he or she achieves good literal understanding, which is the basis for all understanding and comprehension during reading. Unfortunately, awareness of the nature of these basic skills is not well understood. However, with today's easy-to-use eye-movement recording techniques, these skills can be easily evaluated, and today's web-based fluency in silent practice techniques can offer immediate remediation.

QUESTIONS THAT COULD ARISE AFTER READING THIS CHAPTER

1. Why is eye-movement recording not more widely used in all reading diagnosis as the basis for the foundation for remediation?
2. Why is the development of visual and perceptual skills not considered in today's core reading programs?
3. Which students are most likely to require eye-movement recording and how often should they be tested?
4. How can a reading remediation program make the judgment that the techniques employed were successful, without evaluating the changes that were accomplished in a student's Fundamental Reading Process?

Chapter 2

SIGNIFICANCE OF EYE MOVEMENTS

The question is often asked: Do poor eye movements cause poor reading or are they a result of inefficient thought processes? Brandt (1945) stated, "Theoretically, as well as practically, one encounters innumerable difficulties in ascribing a relative degree of cause and effect to respective media of a process. However, in ascribing to the receptor and the effector mutual interdependence, one is not likely to lose sight of or underestimate the importance of the sensory channel in presenting subject matter to the individual, or to underestimate the importance of the motor responses in conscious activity."

One theory holds that poor central processes are due, in part, to inefficient eye-movement habits, and that special training in eye movements would result in more efficient reading.

The other school of thought contends that eye-movement habits are not the cause of the particular mental activity, but rather that central processes determine the characteristic nature of the eye movements themselves.

A third point of view would naturally imply that there exists a functional relationship between ocular movements and central processes. This view recognizes both receptor and effector as a necessary part of the mental equipment to produce what is commonly known as mental activity.

Generally, the position of this author is in agreement with Brandt's statement regarding the mutual interdependence of the receptor and effector, with one point of emphasis. While inefficient central processes can inhibit the development of an efficient oculomotor activity, so can visual/functional and perceptual considerations. For example, a child who suffers from binocular coordination problems could experience many forms of perceptual inaccuracy and physical discomfort to the extent that he or she could never become a truly efficient reader or competent student even though he or she might possess a high level of intelligence.

Although oculomotor activity and the central processes are undoubtedly linked in function and outcome, it is also important to clarify that the influence of both of these processes is not immediate or instantaneous, and thus the effect of one function on the other is rather indirect and can occur after a lapse of time.

Thus it is this author's position that a subject's eye movements, or oculomotor patterns, reflect an acquired reading performance that represents his or her visual/functional, perceptual, and information-processing adaptations over a period of time. The ideal process is described by Anderson and Dearborn (1952) in terms of advanced readers reading at perhaps 500 or more words per minute to "process words rapidly, sequentially, and efficiently without the need for higher-level cognitive functions to interrupt the routine oculomotor activity to any great extent." Further, Radach, Reilly, and Inhoff (2007) emphasize that, "Eye movements are not just an indication of cognition; they are part of the visual processing in reading."

NATURE OF EYE MOVEMENTS

First, it is important to realize that eye movements themselves are not greatly subject to conscious control; therefore the eye movement of an oculomotor pattern that is recorded will, under conditions of reasonable comprehension, be truly reflective of a reader's present level of visual and perceptual efficiency in reading.

There are a number of studies that have shown the relatively involuntary quality of eye movements in various reading and study situations. The comment by Carmichael and Dearborn (1947) aptly summarizes the thought on this subject: ". . . the normal reader cannot 'voluntarily' control the number of his fixation pauses, regressive movements, or the other regular actions of his eyes as he reads. It is possible by very specific training to change the frequency and character of such movements, but this is not accomplished merely by 'consciously trying' to do so. It was not possible, that is, for any subject with whom we have worked to change his eye movements merely by resolving to himself, 'I will now fixate less frequently than I have done in the past and make fewer regressive movements while I carefully read for comprehension this printed page.' This normal subject, of course, has no direct knowledge of the number of fixation pauses or regressive movements that his eyes make as he reads."

Furthermore, the vast majority of readers do not vary their eye-movement performance greatly when reading different types of prose. Seibert (1943) studied the effect of varying subject matter on reading performance. Ballantine (1951), Litterer (1932), Morse (1951), and Taylor, Frackenpohl, and Pettee (1959) studied the effect on reading performance of varying difficulty of content. All of these studies bear out the existence of habits of oculomotor performance in reading and show that the average reader alters his or her eye-movement pattern only slightly, unless the material is far too difficult. This is not to say that oculomotor performance cannot be varied, but research does indicate that the majority of readers perform somewhat characteristically, unless the comprehension demands are unusual or extraordinary.

It is also important to know that a reader will tend to perform, while his or her eye movements are being recorded, in a manner that is quite similar to the manner in which he or she performs while reading a book. Undoubtedly, this is due to the involuntary quality of many of the visual/functional skills and habitual perceptual adaptations involved in reading.

Gilbert and Gilbert (1942) tested 47 fifth-grade pupils to determine whether their reading differed when reading on an eye-movement camera. They found that both comprehension and reading time were not significantly different on the camera and away from it. Tinker (1931) came to the same conclusions from correlations of .87 and .90 between rate and comprehension before and away from the camera. Hoffman, Wellman, and Carmichael (1939), in comparing electrical and photographic recordings of eye movements, also confirmed the fact that people read similarly on and away from an eye-movement camera.

Today with the Visagraph system of recording oculomotor behavior in which a subject's head is not restrained in any way and in which the reading is in a conventional book format, there can be little doubt that a subject's usual or "true" manner of reading is being recorded as seen in Figure 2.1.

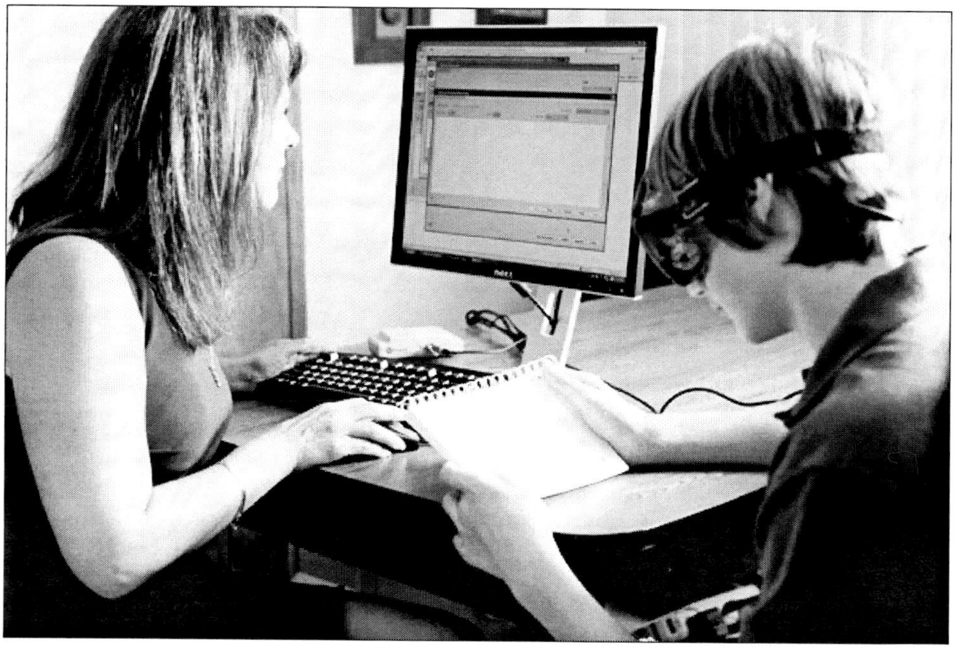

Figure 2.1

It is also important to recognize that an eye-movement recording is primarily a reflection of reading performance and not of achievement (though obviously all factors of the individual's reading development influence achievement test performance). Eye-movement recording provides us with a way of measuring the efficiency with which a person reads through an analysis of objective and measurable components, which comprise what is best termed, according to this author, the Fundamental Reading Process.

An individual's Fundamental Reading Process, as reflected in his or her oculomotor performance, is characterized by the following measurable components in eye-movement recording:

- Fixations–number of eye pauses/100 words
- Regressions–number of reverse eye movements/100 words
- Average Span of Recognition–average number of words or word parts perceived during a fixation
- Average Duration of Fixation–average length of time of eye pause to perceive
- Rate with Comprehension–words per minute read in relation to time
- Directional Attack–tendency to read in a left-to-right manner

Norms for these components were collected in a study by S. E. Taylor (1960) involving over 12,000 students in grades one through college level throughout the United States and are shown in the following table.

Table 2.1

Table National Norms														Advanced				
Grade Level	**1**	**2**	**3**	**4**	**5**	**6**	**7**	**8**	**9**	**10**	**11**	**12**	**Col.**	**1**	**2**	**3**	**4**	**5**
Fixations/100 Words	224	174	155	139	129	120	114	109	105	101	96	94	90	77	65	57	48	44
Regressions/100 Words	52	40	35	31	28	25	23	21	20	19	18	17	15	11	8	5	4	2
Directional Attack %	23	23	23	24	22	21	20	19	19	19	19	18	17	14	12	9	8	5
Av. Span of Recognition	.45	.57	.65	.72	.78	.83	.88	.92	.95	.99	1.04	1.06	1.11	1.30	1.53	1.75	2.08	2.27
Av. Duration of Fixation	.33	.30	.28	.27	.27	.27	.27	.27	.27	.26	.26	.25	.24	.23	.23	.22	.22	.22
WPM Rate w/Comprehension	80	115	138	158	173	185	195	204	214	224	237	250	280	340	400	480	560	620

Levels 1 - College—Taken from "Grade Level Norms for the Components of the Fundamental Reading Skill," by Stanford E. Taylor, Helen Frackenpohl, and James L. Pettee, EDL Research and Information Bulletin No. 3, Educational Developmental Laboratories, Inc., 1960.
Advanced—Represents typical reading performance characteristics for trained readers, accumulated from various reading centers employing instrument training techniques and using eye-movement photography as an evaluative procedure.

You might think of eye-movement recording as a time-and-motion study of the reading process that can allow one to make judgments about certain aspects of a student's silent reading ability.

- Ease and comfort–Does reading appear to be a visually coordinated and a comfortable activity?
- Energy–Is the student reading in an expeditious manner, with an appropriate amount of visual activity to complete the reading task?
- Time–Can the student read at adequate rates, completing reading tasks in a reasonable period of time?
- Effectiveness–Does the reader read in a manner that is orderly in terms of perception, and process information in a manner that facilitates retention and comprehension?
- Enjoyment–Has reading developed into an efficient process that will encourage habits of recreational reading?

FORMATION OF AN OCULOMOTOR BEHAVIOR

Individuals acquire their Fundamental Reading Process skills and the oculomotor activity they employ in reading during beginning reading as they make a series of vision-related, as well as visual/functional, perceptual, and information processing adjustments. An individual's oculomotor development and its refinement begins during the earliest days, when a child directs his or her eyes in "looking" activities and then tries to apply these general observation habits to the near point task of reading.

Key points to note with regard to oculomotor development are:

- Trial-and-error learning
- "Looking" activities
- Vision, binocular coordination, etc.

By school age children have already formed pronounced oculomotor habits. A longitudinal study by Taylor and Robinson (1963) involving eye-movement photography confirmed that children enter kindergarten or first grade with established oculomotor habits born out of their cumulative preschool looking experiences. Perhaps the most distinctive of these habits is the tendency of children to move their eyes quite frequently, despite variations in the material being viewed or the task assigned. Children tend to move their eyes over visual material at a rate of three movements per second, thus pausing rather habitually for an average duration of .33 seconds.

As the children in the study began to read, it was apparent that this habitual .33 of a second duration in eye pause was not adequate for identification and recognition of a word, for all of the children resorted to making an average of two or three fixations for every word encountered. This "stalling" or moving about a word is not easily recognized and is quite characteristic of beginning readers (of any age) and is most excessive with individuals with more serious learning disabilities.

Other key points to note regarding oculomotor behavior are:

- Basal word load in first-year reading contributes to non-fluent reading behaviors
- Vision, binocular coordination, etc. contribute to the manner in which students move accurately across print during reading

Indeed if one looks at national averages for the number of fixations and regressions per 100 words in the norm chart by Taylor, Frackenpohl, and Pettee (1960), it would seem that the traditional "learning to read" word recognition experiences and visual discrimination training have not proved sufficient to eliminate the need for multiple fixations per word. Nor do the usual verbal directions given to encourage effective directional attack appear successful when one considers the persistent and numerous regressions that occur in the eye-movement records of the majority of beginning readers.

Consider that in a typical first-year beginning reading program, children are introduced to perhaps 350 to 800 new words. Unless sufficient word recognition automaticity ("flash" practice) is provided, the resulting quantity of new words encountered each week in basal reading or "whole language" reading approaches will continuously condition non-fluent reading behaviors characterized by an excessive number of fixations and regressions and prolonged duration of fixation. Perhaps, too, a child may be handicapped by imperfect vision, inadequate binocular coordination, or problems with fusion or motility. These impediments will result in a less precise and efficient visual process and, as such, will inhibit the perceptual process.

It is important to realize that reading is not a normal human visual activity, but one that must be learned. A considerable number of children do not typically possess adequate binocular coordination, ocular motility, or accuracy in tracking across lines of print. A lack of visual/functional competence can make reading uncomfortable and result in poorer word perception, which increases the number of fixations and regressions per word during reading.

Additional problems to note are:

- Oral reading
- Overstress on phonics
- Comprehension difficulty
- Lack of confidence

According to the results of a study by Gilbert (1940), round-robin oral reading can also encourage and condition an excessive number of random ocular movements as children follow along in their books while another child reads slowly and laboriously. Even the act of oral reading by a given student on his or her own reading performance can result in random fixations since the time to "see and say" usually exceeds the usual fixation time of one-third of a second.

An overstress on phonics in primary grades can cause some children to analyze words compulsively. This results in a tendency to analyze and vocalize most words read. Such an overstress on phonics will limit the development of fluency in silent reading and can also result in an inadequate oculomotor activity in later grades.

Should the child also experience unusual difficulty with comprehension, experience social ridicule when attempting oral reading, or lack the necessary confidence in his or her own ability to read, the result can be an unsatisfactory adjustment to the reading act, and can take the form of tremors in eye-movements, excessive head movement, blinking, random ocular movements, and an excessive number of fixations and regressions.

And so, as children struggle with word identification and recognition and to understand what they read, they are not, in most beginning reading procedures today, provided with an opportunity to develop any great amount of efficiency in the way they read. To the contrary, the beginning reader is subjected to a variety of situations and influences, which condition a perceptual and oculomotor behavior that is characterized by an excessive number of fixations and regressions, a restricted span of recognition, and a prolonged duration of fixation. This position is based on comparisons of eye-movement recordings of students before and after reading improvement programs that are designed to correct and compensate for the lack of proper visual/functional and perceptual training in the early grades. Taylor (1966) describes and presents many eye-movement photographs of the changes that can be effected by various forms of perceptual training. Likewise, this author (1976–1978) has reported on changes in eye-movement behaviors achieved by developmental and corrective reading programs that utilize reading instrumentation to develop fluency in reading as part of the reading curriculum.

CONCLUSION

During their early reading experiences, all readers will develop an oculomotor activity that is not subject to great variation. This acquired reading performance activity can be easily and accurately evaluated through today's eye-movement recording techniques, and this would lead to a better defined program of reading fluency development.

QUESTIONS THAT COULD ARISE AFTER READING THIS CHAPTER

1. What should be the logical goals in terms of oculomotor development for different readers in different grades and levels of reading competency?
2. Since oculomotor activity is such a key consideration in relation to fluency in silent reading, why has reading performance examination not been incorporated into testing of all students who are experiencing difficulty in reading?
3. What changes in beginning reading need to be incorporated to ensure the development of an efficient oculomotor activity in reading?

This chapter also raises questions as to how best to embrace computer technology to develop many of the high-speed processes of silent reading. While a teacher can and should continue with those instructional areas that require student/teacher interaction (such as introduction of reading vocabulary, phonics guidance, direction of reading comprehension goals and strategies, and appreciation of literary content), it would seem logical that computer technology must also be provided to students to ensure the development of the more fundamental visual/perceptual skills that function three to five times per second.

Chapter 3

HISTORY OF EYE MOVEMENT RECORDING

Since the first studies of eye movements by Javal (1879), a multitude of ingenious methods have been used in an effort to learn more about how our eyes serve us. The following list gives some idea of the evolution of these methods, from the stage of direct observation through the development of mechanical and electrical devices for recording eye movements to the more refined stage of photography, and finally, to electronic sensing of eye movements. In describing here the various methods of recording eye movements, the author made an attempt to include a representative sampling of each broad category. Those interested in a more complete history of earlier developments would do well to consult Carmichael and Dearborn (1947), Taylor (1937), and Yarbus (1967).

Direct Observation

- A mirror was placed either beside or above the reading material so that an observer could count eye movements by watching the subject's eyes (Freeman, 1916; Javal, 1879).
- Telescopes, microscopes, magnifying lenses, and other means to magnify the eye were used so that the observer could more clearly see and count eye movements (Barany, 1920, George, Toren, & Lowell, 1923; Morse, 1951).
- A small peephole was cut into the middle of the copy to be read. The observer peered through this hole to count the eye movements made by the subject (Miles, 1928).

All of these methods of direct observation have similar failings–the observer is unable to notice and/or remember many of the more rapid and subtle movements (in any direct observation method, from one-quarter to one-half of the movements will be missed, varying with the observer); the movements cannot be evaluated at a later date on a qualitative basis; and obviously no oculomotor pattern could be studied or appreciated.

Mechanical

- Levers were placed against the side of the eyeball or fastened directly to the eyelid with adhesive tape. As the eye rotated, the movements were amplified through additional levers, and the movements were recorded on smoked paper (Ohm, 1914).
- Pneumatic capsules were laid over the eyelid or against the eyeball. The movement of the eye compressed the capsule, which activated a tambour, and this in turn activated a recording stylus (Buys, 1910 to 1911).
- A tambour with a protruding stem was held against one eyeball. Two rubber tubes running from the tambour were inserted into the ears of the experimenter. The changes in air pressure were audible, allowing the experimenter to listen to and count the movements (Lamare, 1892).
- Cups made of ivory, aluminum, rubber, and other materials were form-fitted to the cornea. Attached to the cups were levels of threads, which activated a recording stylus when the eye moved. Another experimenter placed a mirror on the cup, which reflected a beam of light onto a screen where the movements could be observed (Ahren, 1891, Delabarre, 1898, Huey, 1898).

The more sophisticated use of cups attached to the eye was introduced by Yarbus in 1956 in Moscow, as shown in Figure 3.1. Suction cups that deflected light rays to record eye-movement positions (P1) and cups that control the nature of images falling on the retina (P8) were among the eight different types of cups designed by Yarbus (1967).

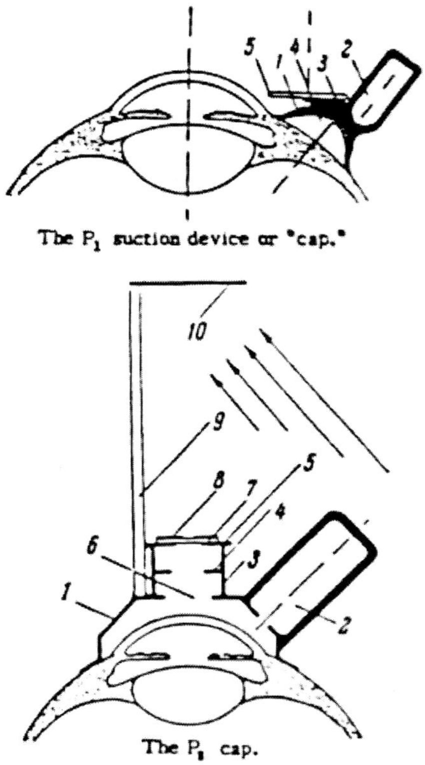

Figure 3.1

Electrical

- The pneumatic capsule was again used to activate a tambour, and its movement was used to break an electrical circuit, transferring the changes in air pressure into sound. The experimenter counted fixations by listening (Lamare, 1892).
- Electrodes, as shown in Figure 3.2, were attached around the eyes of the subject, and the small amount of electric current generated by moving the eye was received, amplified, and recorded with an ink-writing oscillograph (Carmichael & Dearborn, 1947).

While the electrode method was superior to all previously mentioned techniques, and was undoubtedly more sensitive, its primary disadvantage lay in its electrical complexity and the careful technical control needed to maintain an accurate recording. As a research tech-

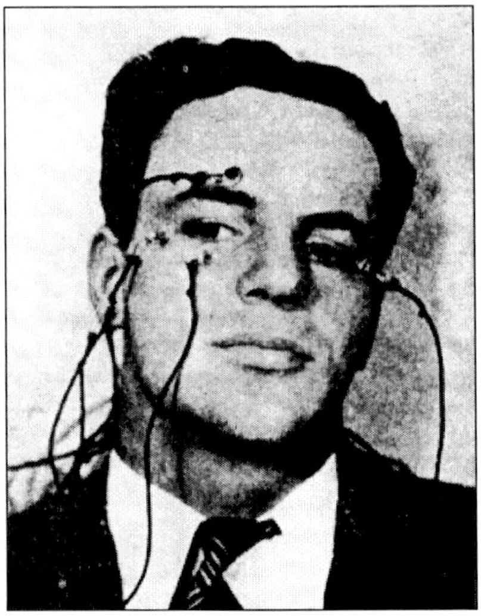

Figure 3.2

nique, however, this method had certain advantages over many other methods in that the subject's eyes were unencumbered and the head was relatively free.

Photographic

- Small pieces or flakes of Chinese white pigment were placed on the cornea of the eye, and a motion picture camera photographed the full face of the subject, as shown in Figure 3.3. The motion pictures were enlarged through projection, and the movement of the "eye-spot" plotted off to indicate the movement of the eye (Judd, McAllister, & Steele, 1905).
- A mirror was mounted into a spectacle frame so that it could be held against a closed eyelid, as shown in Figure 3.4. A bead of light was reflected from the mirror and recorded onto photographic film.

This optical frame was designed by Dr. Raymond Dodge (1907). Later, this frame was adapted by Roland C. Travis (1932) for monocular recording of eye movements.

With the kinetoscopic method, there were obvious limitations to the ease with which the pigment could be applied and caused to remain in place. In addition, the bead recorded was too gross to reveal ocular

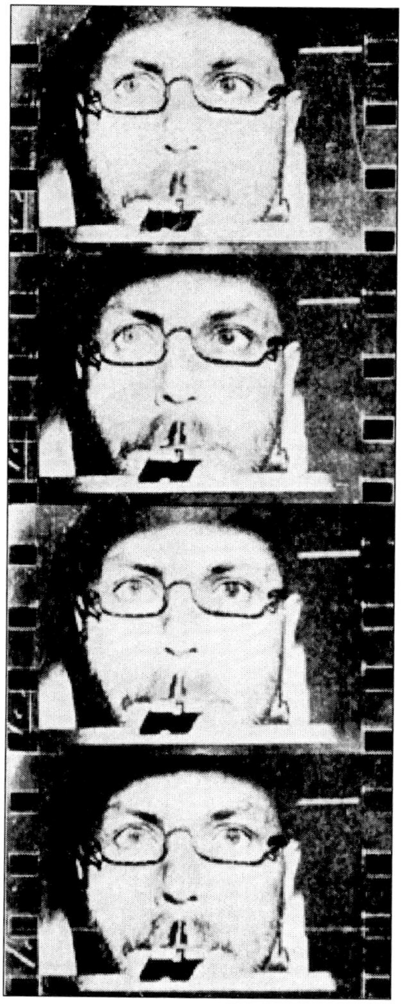

Figure 3.3

movement subtleties. Then, too, it was an extremely long and difficult task to project the photographs in order to trace the beads. The disadvantage of the mirror reflection method is that the two eyes are not used in reading as they would normally be, plus the fact that the mirror reflection could not accurately reflect all of the subtleties of eye movements.

- Beads from sidelights were shown onto the cornea of the eyes, producing a corneal reflection, which was photographed through lenses of specially designed cameras onto constantly moving motion picture film.

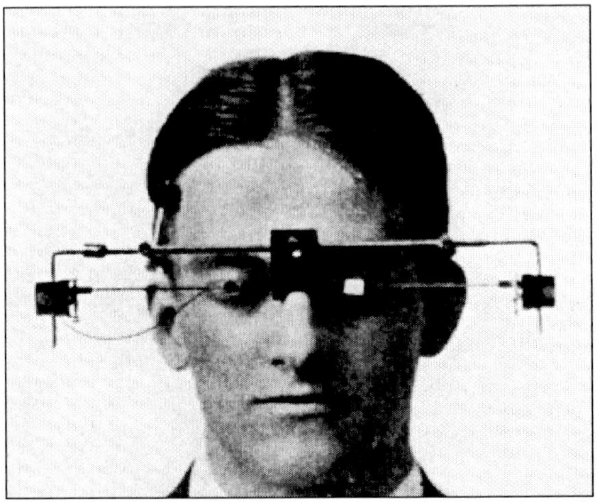

Figure 3.4

The corneal reflection method proved to be more practical than all prior methods of recording and became the most widely used method for studying eye movements through the 1960s. Dr. Raymond Dodge (1907), the first to use this method, called attention to the fact that the amplitude of movement of the reflection was equal to one-half of the actual displacement of the apex of the cornea, but was always in the same direction. Used in recording eye movements in reading, this corneal slippage is of no real significance and does not in any way obscure the movements or detract from the accuracy of the recording.

From 1899 through the 1930s, many corneal reflection cameras were built at various universities for educational and psychological research. A number of these cameras are pictured here. Most of the illustrations on the following pages depicting the early stages of eye-movement recording are taken from *Controlled Reading* by E. A. Taylor (1937). Also pictured is the Ophthalmograph, the first eye-movement camera commercially available in the United States. The Reading Eye, developed by this author in 1959, was the most widely used development in corneal reflection photography.

1. The Wesleyan University Camera, designed by Dr. Raymond Dodge between 1899 and 1901, was known as the "falling-plate," or Dodge-Cline camera, and is shown in Figure 3.5. This was the first camera to use the corneal reflection method (Dodge & Cline, 1901).

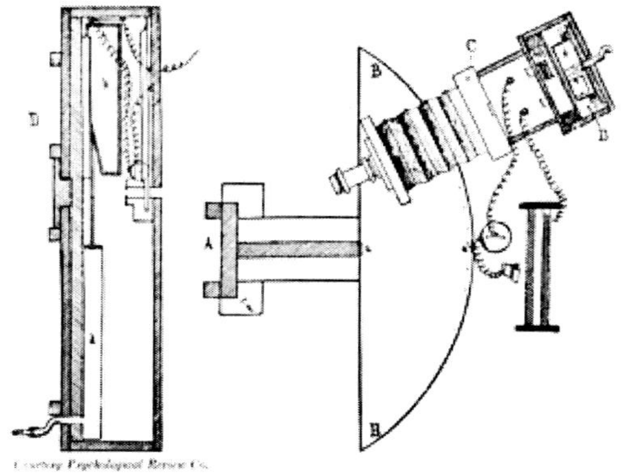

Figure 3.5

2. The Columbia University Camera was built by Dr. Walter Dearborn, partially under the direction of Dr. Dodge between 1903 and 1904. This camera, shown in Figure 3.6, was used to secure the first systematic study of eye movements in reading (Dearborn, 1906).

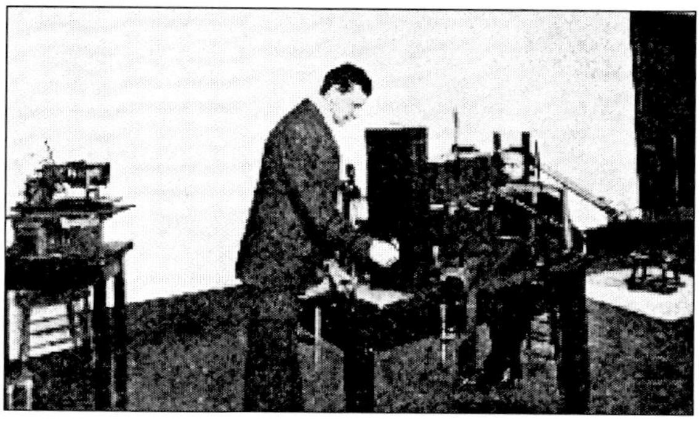

Figure 3.6

3. The University of Wisconsin Camera, an improved camera designed by Dr. Walter F. Dearborn, 1905 to 1907, used a three-inch film approximately three feet long, propelled by a roller friction drive as shown in Figure 3.7.

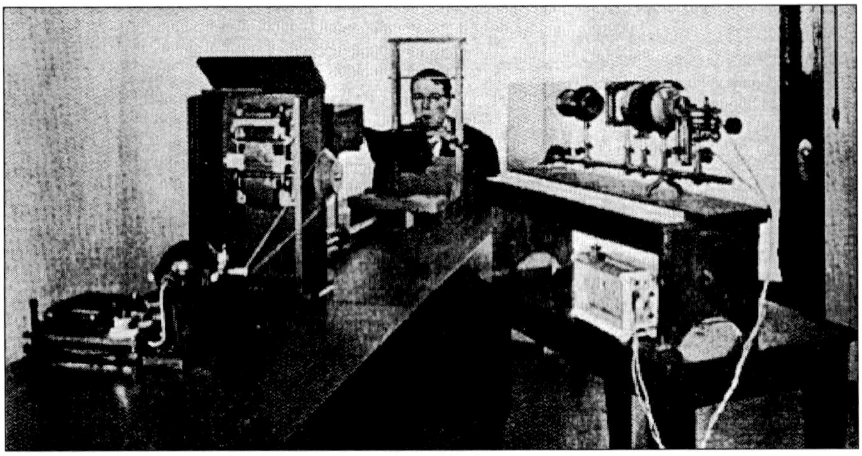

Figure 3.7

4. The University of Chicago Camera, designed by Dr. Clarence T. Gray between 1910 and 1911 (Gray, 1917), and improved and modified by Dr. Guy T. Buswell (1935), is shown in Figure 3.8. This camera provided for binocular photography, as well as photographing a third bead to distinguish head movements, and was the first camera to use motion picture film.

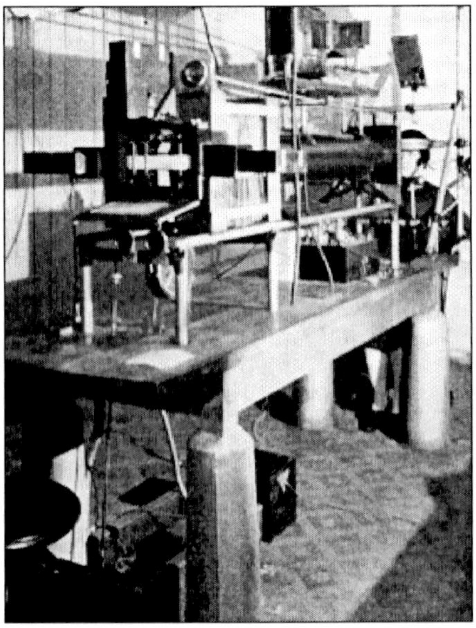

Figure 3.8

5. The Stanford University Camera, designed by Dr. Raymond Dodge and re-modeled by Dr. Walter R. Miles in 1922, is shown in Figure 3.9. This camera used a length of panchromatic film instead of the falling-plate principle and recorded both horizontal and vertical movements (Miles & Shen, 1925).

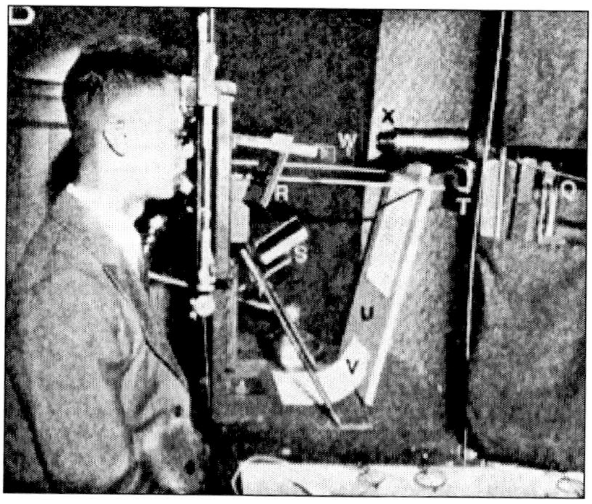

Figure 3.9

6. The University of Texas Camera, shown in Figure 3.10, was designed by Dr. Clarence T. Gray between 1913 and 1914 (Gray 1917), and later remodeled by Dr. B. F. Holland (1927).

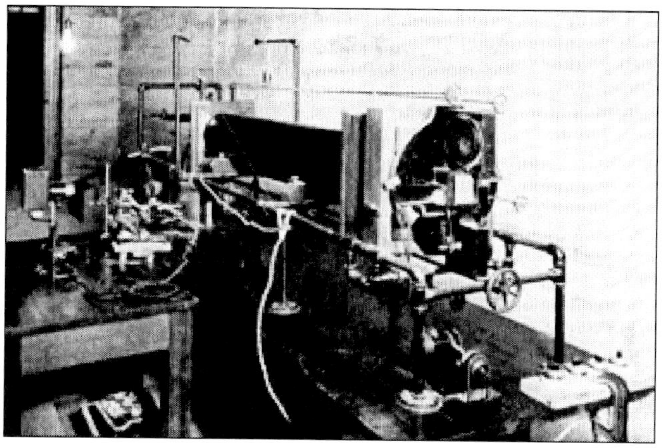

Figure 3.10

7. The University of Cambridge Camera, designed by M. D. Vernon in 1928 (Vernon 1930), is shown in Figure 3.11.

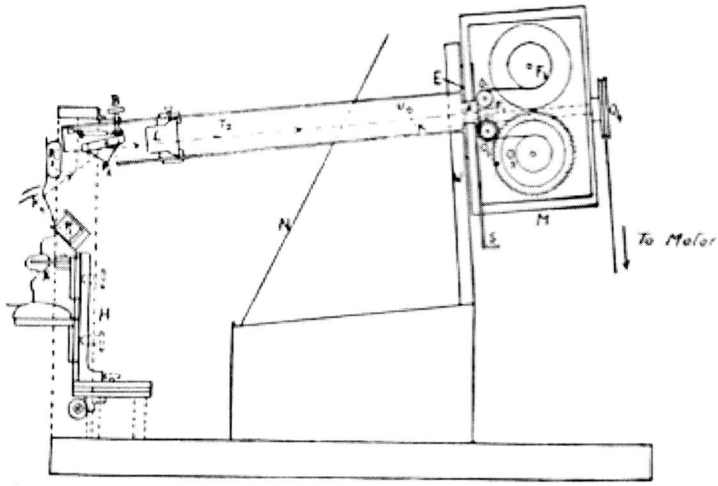

Figure 3.11

8. The Optokinetograph at Harvard University, as shown in Figure 3.12, was built under the direction of Dr. Walter F. Dearborn in 1929.

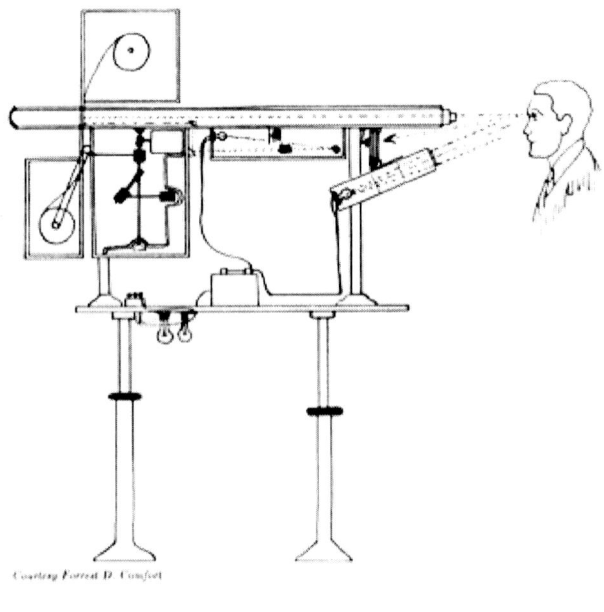

Figure 3.12

9. The University of Nebraska Camera, as shown in Figure 3.13, was built by Dr. J. P. Guilford, and was an improvement over those he had built at Cornell University and the University of Kansas in 1929 (Guilford & Hackman, 1936).

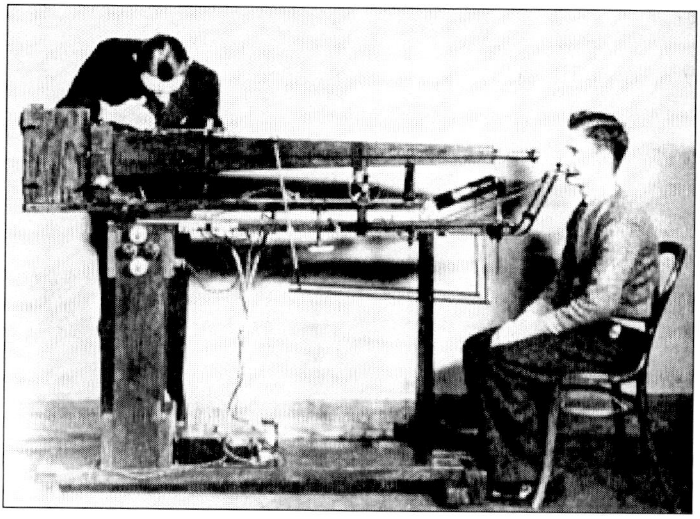

Figure 3.13

10. The University of Minnesota Camera, as shown in Figure 3.14, was built under the direction of Dr. Miles A. Tinker in 1931. This is one of the most elaborate of the large cameras constructed (Tinker, 1931).

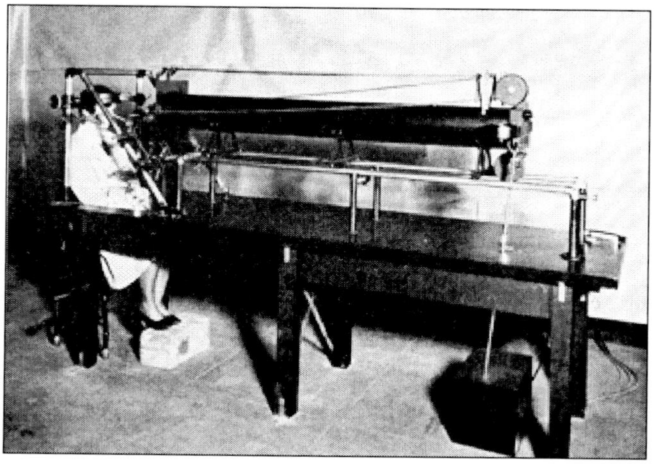

Figure 3.14

11. The first portable monocular eye-movement camera built by James Y. Taylor and Carl C. Taylor of Educational Laboratories, Brownwood, Texas, in 1932, is shown in Figure 3.15.

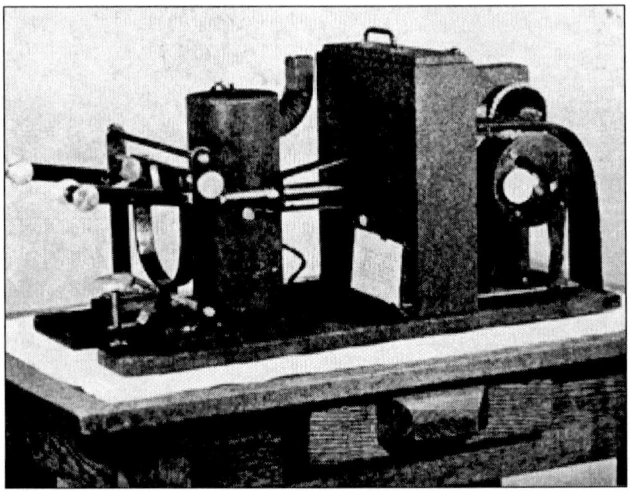

Figure 3.15

12. The Ophthalmograph, shown in Figure 3.16, was designed by James Y. Taylor, Carl C. Taylor, and Earl A. Taylor in 1932. This portable binocular camera was distributed by American Optical Company until 1939.

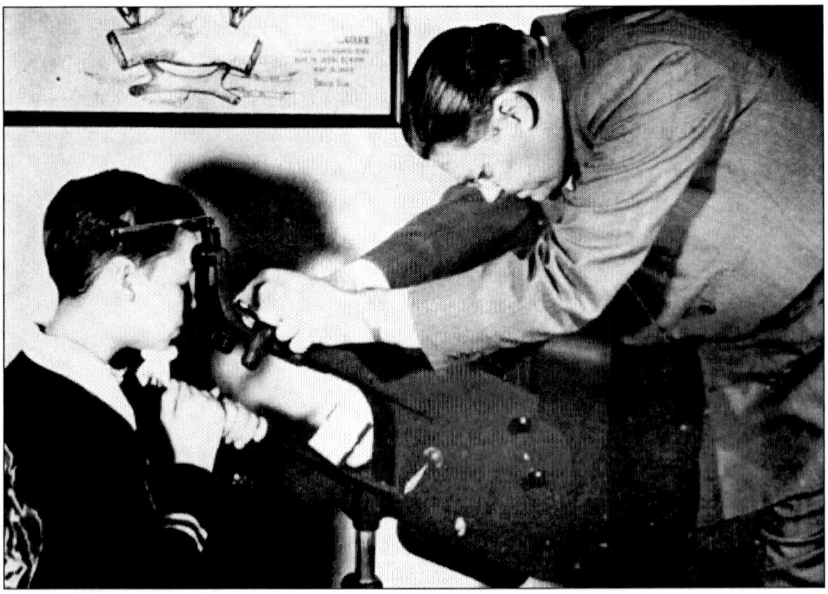

Figure 3.16

13. The University of Chicago Camera, shown in Figure 3.17, was built under the direction of Dr. Guy T. Buswell in 1933. This camera recorded both horizontal and vertical eye movements on two separate films to study the perception of art (Buswell, 1935).

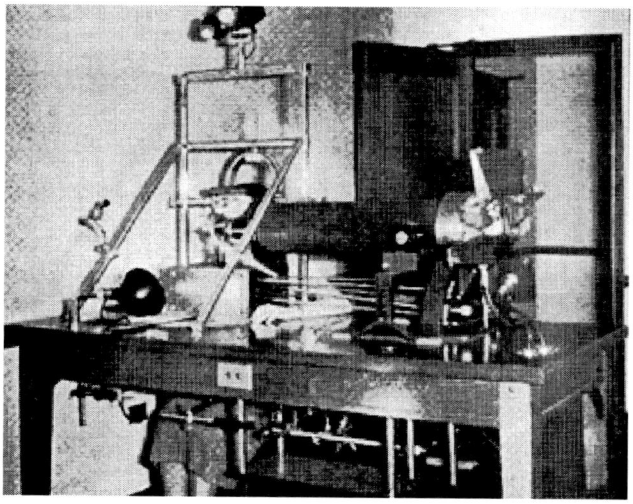

Figure 3.17

14. A small portable eye-movement camera built at the University of Chicago by Dr. Buswell in 1935 is shown in Figure 3.18.

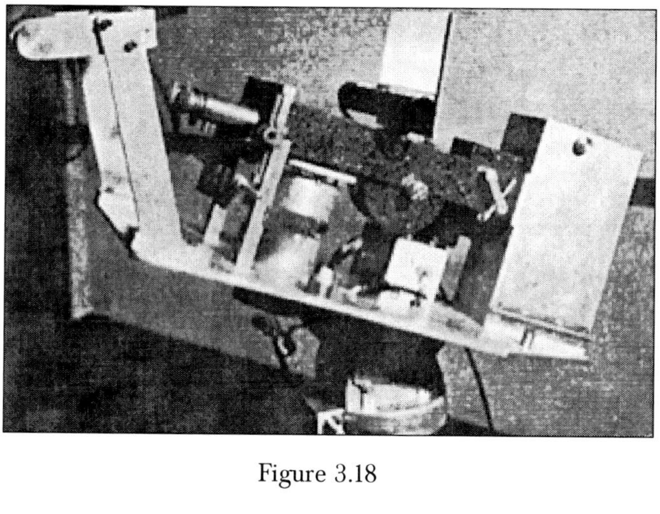

Figure 3.18

15. In the 1960s, the Reading Eye I, as shown in Figure 3.19, was released by S. E. Taylor.

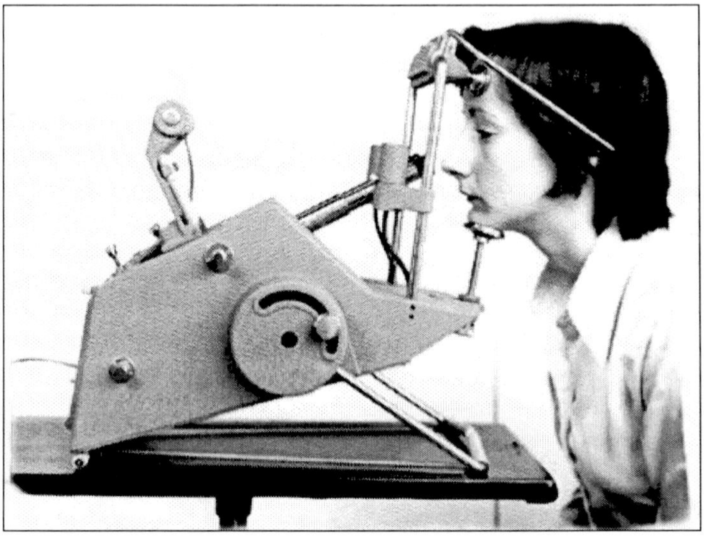

Figure 3.19

16. In the late 1960s, head cameras, such as that developed by Mackworth and shown in Figure 3.20, were used to record eye movements. Usually such cameras were used only in general observation situations as contrasted to that of reading.

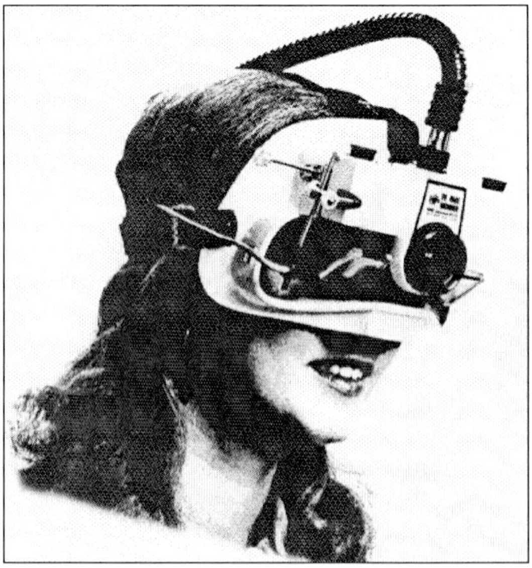

Figure 3.20

Electronic

- Reflections of the limbus of the eye projected on photo diodes sensed changes in eye-movement positions producing variations in electrical voltage. These voltage changes were amplified and used in conjunction with heated pen recordings.
- TV cameras were employed to photograph eye movements.
- Reflections of the change in limbus positions were translated into varying voltages, which in turn were recorded as digital information by computers.

The Reading Eye II (or Eye Trac) became one of the more widely used and commercially available means of measuring eye movements during the 1970s.

- The Reading Eye II (or Eye Trac), as shown in Figure 3.21, was produced by Applied Science Laboratories of Waltham, Massachusetts (Morris, 1973).

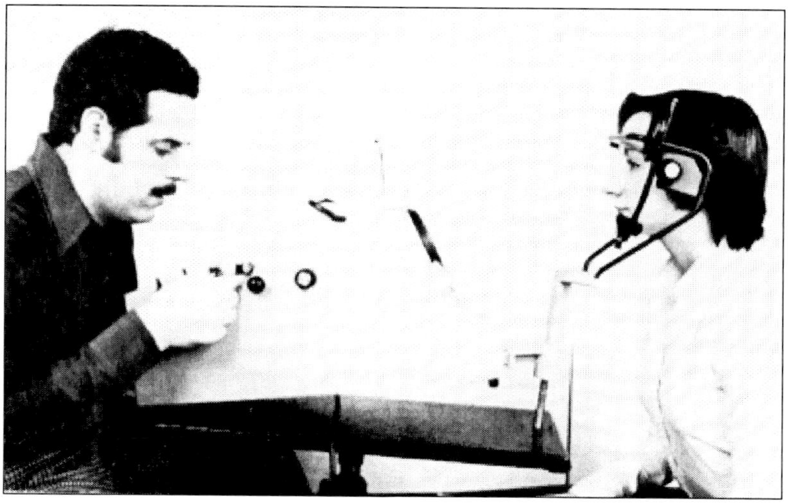

Figure 3.21

- TV recording of eye movements was also employed, as shown in Figure 3.22.

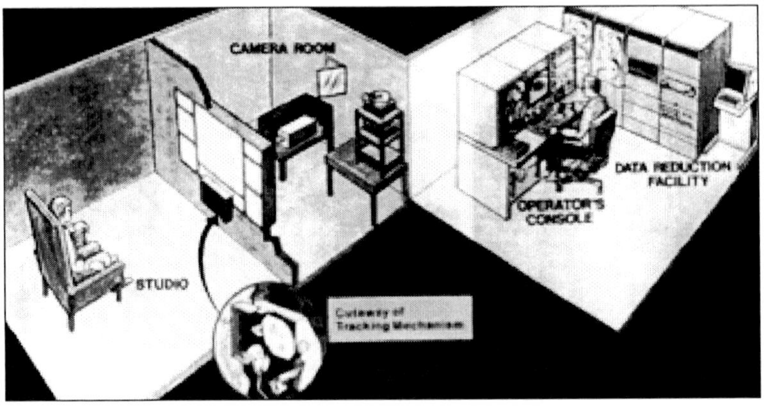

Figure 3.22

Computerized Recordings

Computerized recordings, introduced during the late 1970s, were used principally in research situations to study such factors as the nature of the oculomotor activity, the span of recognition, and the effect of context on oculomotor behavior.

These studies are most comprehensively covered by Rayner (1983) in his publication *Eye Movements in Reading: Perceptual and Language Processes.*

A Dual Purkinja Image Eyetracker, developed by SRI International, as shown in Figure 3.23, was used at the University of Illinois by Dr. George W. McConkie in his studies of eye-movement behavior and the reading process. This equipment tracks two of four reflections from different structures in the eye, sampling the eye's position 1,000 times per second.

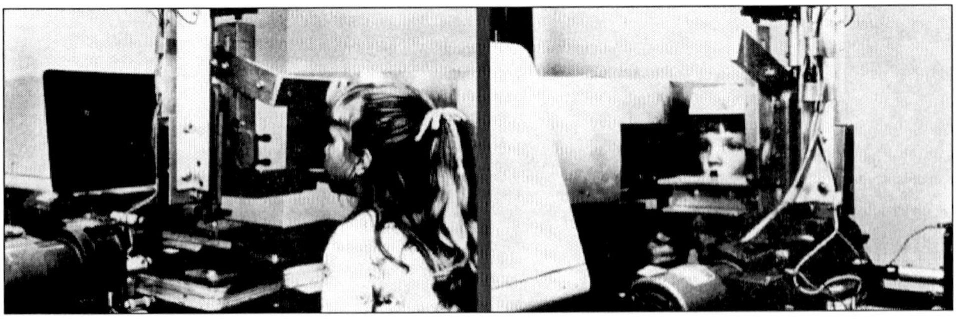

Figure 3.23

The Visagraph I, designed by this author and shown in Figure 3.24, was released during 1985 and was the first eye-movement recording system in schools to employ the microcomputer as a means of recording and analyzing oculomotor performance during reading. It combined the ease and accuracy of electronic sensing and recording with the flexibility, extensive memory, and analytical capability of the computer.

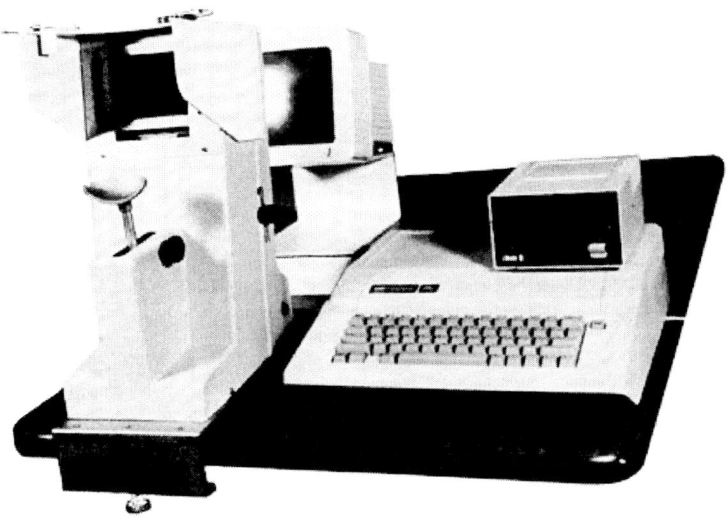

Figure 3.24

The introduction of the Visagraph II, with the advancements and accuracy of its recording and the amount of information that could be determined in comparison to past eye-movement recording systems, opened up new vistas of testing and research.

The advantage of Visagraph II was in the use of goggles (shown in Figure 3.25) containing infrared sensors that eliminate the effects of head movement and also removes the need for calibration and alignment for each subject. As with the Visagraph II, the Visagraph III automatically calculates reading efficiency components and provides graphs of a subject's reading performance.

The Visagraph III produces both a Reading Report (reading performance characteristics) and a Visual/Functional Report (visual coordination and visual/functional performances). The Visagraph III is the most widely used eye-movement recording device today. As of 2012, there are over 2,000 Visagraph III eye-movement recording devices used by schools, clinics, and vision specialists.

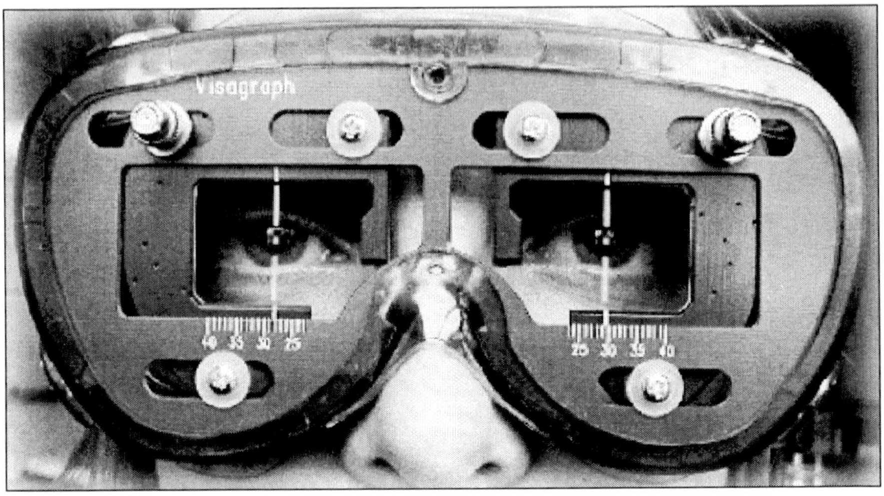

Figure 3.25

Chapter 4

USING THE VISAGRAPH EYE MOVEMENT RECORDING SYSTEM

This chapter will explain the process of eye-movement recording and the nature of the findings that can help determine which reading fluency development techniques would be effective training practice activities.

WHO TO RECORD

Consider that Every Student Deserves a Visagraph Examination

You might consider using the Visagraph to determine which students are most in need of silent reading fluency development practice.

If time permits, a school's entire student body should receive a Visagraph eye-movement appraisal. After review of all appraisals, the students who should be scheduled first for fluency development are those whose reading performances (in terms of fixations and regressions) are greater than grade-level norms and whose reading rate is less than the 35 percent of the rate goal for a given level.

Many schools will also use the Visagraph as a screening technique to ensure that students' reading fluency is up to par as they advance to more demanding study requirements. The most critical points in determining when eye-movement recording should be used are as follows:

- Grade 3–to ensure that students possess a reasonable level of reading efficiency as preparation for the more extensive and complex test-type reading and study activities they will encounter in the intermediate grades.

A reasonable goal at this point would be a reading rate equal to or in excess of 180 words per minute (beyond the usual oral rate range), with commensurate efficiency in terms of oculomotor characteristics.

- Grade 6–to ensure that students' reading efficiency levels are sufficient to prepare them for the more extensive reading study and research tasks they will face at the secondary level. Furthermore, high levels of reading fluency are essential for truly effective skimming and scanning activities, which students should engage in at the secondary level to be truly effective in their studies.

A desirable goal at this point would be a reading rate at or in excess of 270 words per minute with accompanying efficiency in terms of oculomotor characteristics.

- Grade 11 (college bound)–again, to ensure that students who are college bound are prepared for the more extensive reading tasks they will encounter in their advanced studies.

A reading rate deemed suitable for the amount of assigned reading at the college level would seem to be 300 to 400 words per minute with accompanying appropriate oculomotor efficiency.

- Adults (any level)–to determine that adults possess the reading efficiency necessary to perform their job responsibilities. Once a survey of reading level needs has been conducted (typically ninth level or higher), eye-movement recording can be employed to determine whether an individual's reading efficiency is sufficient or in accord with that reading level expectation.

SELECTING THE APPROPRIATE READING TEST LEVEL

The Visagraph Test Booklet contains 48 test selections for grades 1 through 12 all measured using The Lexile® Framework for Reading, as shown in the following table.

Table 4.1

All measured using The Lexile® Framework for Reading.

Grade	Estimated Lexile measures
1	300L
2	570L
3	750L
4	810L
5	850L
6	960L
7	1010L
8	1110L
9	1140L
10	1170L
11	1200L
12	1230L

Ideally, the level of a reading test selection should be at a subject's Independent Reading Level (IRL) or slightly lower. It is important that a subject read a very easy-to-read test selection during eye-movement recording to exhibit a characteristic and continuous reading performance. Only when the reading content is read easily and independently can the examiner be assured that the subject's reading performance is typical of the most fluent manner of reading possible.

Use of an Oral Pretest

Whenever there is doubt concerning a subject's ability to read selections even at Level 1, or sometimes as a means for confirming the appropriateness of a given level of test content, an oral pretest can be administered prior to recording. For this purpose, the examiner will use the Visagraph Test Selection Booklet. He or she would introduce a selection by saying, "This is a story about . . . Would you read this story to me?" The purpose of this introduction is to ensure the fact that the subject knows the name of the individual in the test selection or is familiar with the topic of the selection.

The subject would then read orally and the examiner would listen, noting any hesitancy and the number of words that are mispronounced or miscalled. Another reading of a test selection on a lower level is recommended if the subject misses more than 5 percent of the words in a test selection (approximately two to three words for Test Selections Levels 1 through 3, or four to five words on Levels 4 and up).

If a student's independent reading level were already known, a test selection on this level would be used for the oral pretest. If not, a grade level selection would be used first. Adults who have completed high school might begin with a Level 10 high school test selection. Adults who have not completed high school might start with a junior high school test selection, perhaps Level 7.

If a subject reads fluently and with apparent ease, there is no need to complete the reading of the test selection. Perhaps only one or two sentences need be read. If, however, the subject exhibits some degree of hesitancy, it may be best to have the entire selection read in order to make a determination as to whether or not an easier test selection may be more appropriate. If words are miscalled, or if there is extreme hesitance throughout the reading, it may be advisable to ask the subject to read a test selection at the next lower level. This process of sampling reading test selections is continued until the subject can read a certain level of test content with reasonable ease.

Once an appropriate level of test selection has been determined, another test selection at that level would be selected for use in the Visagraph testing routine.

C. INTERPRETING THE READING REPORT

The Reading Report, as shown in Figure 4.1, provides automatic calculations of all reading performance characteristics.

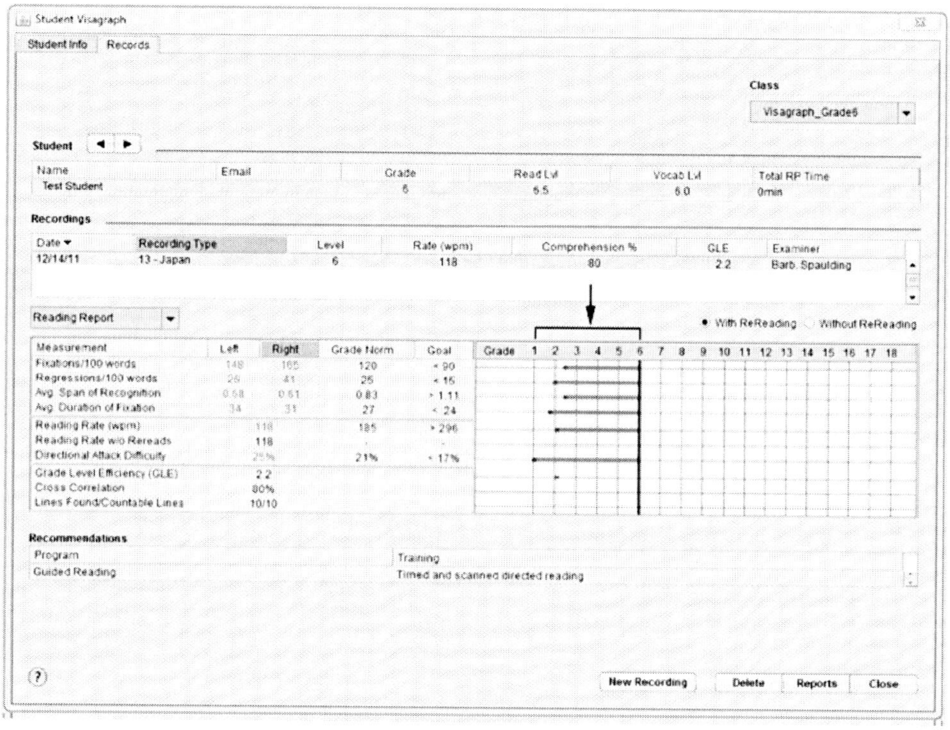

Figure 4.1

Automatic calculations of reading performance characteristics will appear, as well as grade level normative performances and desirable goals. Additionally, there will be a plot of the characteristics of the most active eye against Taylor's National Norms. The shaded area in the report is the most active eye, not necessarily the dominant eye.

Important Considerations

1. The most significant indicator of reading efficiency is a student's Grade Level Efficiency (GLE). These calculations take into account both a student's reading rate as well as the amount of visual activity during reading. Most judgments regarding the need for fluency development will be made on the basis of GLE.
2. Next take note of the number of Fixations and Regressions. At times, a GLE may seem adequate, but a student's high reading rate may still involve too many fixations and regressions, with very short

duration of fixations. This can still indicate a need for fluency development to change the nature of the visual activity of reading to be more in line with a student's reading rate.

3. Then check the Reading Rate with Comprehension (with rereading) against the reading rate without rereading. Ideally, these two rates should be the same, indicating no rereading. If there were rereading, you might consider the reading rate without rereading as more typical. Or, time permitting, rerecord and caution the subject not to reread.
4. Look also at Directional Attack Difficulty. Even if the number of fixations is relatively low, it is important that the percentage of regressions to fixations be relatively low (less than 10 to 15 percent) to indicate proper sequencing of word impressions to short-term memory.
5. Lastly, check Cross Correlation. If very low, perhaps 75 percent or lower, you might consider a retest confirming the student's IPD (interpupillary distance) alignment to ensure a good recording. If the cross correlation is below 90 percent, you might first look at the student's Visual/Functional Report to see if there were any indicators of binocular problems (data in red). You might administer the Student Inventory Questions to further confirm that the low correlation was indicative of visual/functional problems.

If a student's Cross Correlation is low, perhaps 90 percent or lower, there will likely be many indicators in the Visual Functional Report that suggest binocular problems. The student's responses to the Student Inventory Questions will also suggest problems. In this event, the student should logically be referred to a vision specialist for more complete diagnosis.

Nature of Fixations

A fixation or eye stop is that interval in reading during which the eye is held relatively stationary for a brief time, during which perception takes place. Following each fixation, the eye then moves to a new fixation position. This interfixation movement is often called a saccade or saccadic movement, for the eye acts as if it is being thrown or jerked. One set of muscles, termed the agonists, contracts, putting the eye into motion. The eye is brought to a stop when a second set of muscles, the antagonists, contract, producing a relative equilibrium of forces. The eye is never completely still; however, it is sufficiently stationary to allow perception to take place. The eye moves in this fashion across each line of print in a series of fixations or eye stops and then sweeps back in another larger saccadic movement to the beginning of the next line of print, which is commonly referred to as a return sweep.

Figure 4.2 by this author (2011) displays the many functions that occur somewhat concurrently during a fixation following a saccade.

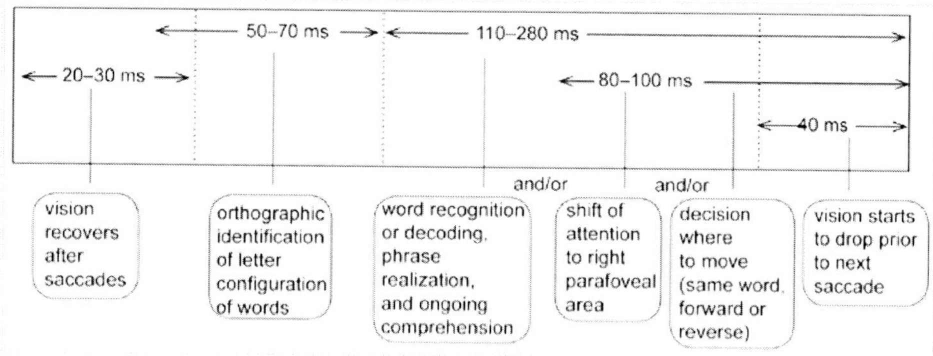

Figure 4.2

Although the interval of suppression of vision during a saccade to a new fixation or regression is debated, it does exist. Further, in a study by Solan, Hansen, Shelley-Tremblay, and Ficarra (2004), students with magnocellular deficit, who did not exhibit normal suppression of vision during saccadic movements, did experience perceptual limitations by virtue of blurred print and overlapping images. Although there seems to be some difference of opinion as to how long a delay occurs before vision returns to normal, it would seem that there is some initial period during a new fixation where vision is suppressed, likely 20 to 30 milliseconds minimally.

During a saccadic movement, as shown in the following illustration, most researchers have concluded that the visual impression is a "smear," and cannot provide sufficient letter awareness that might be meaningful for word recognition.

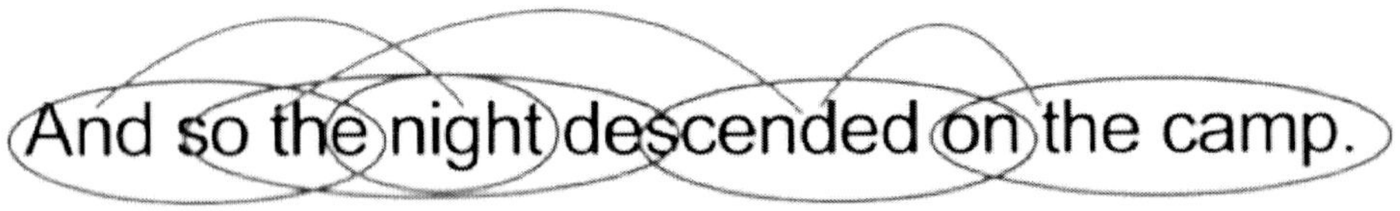

Figure 4.3

The amplitude of saccadic movement to a new fixation would seem to be influenced by a reader's span of recognition, which in turn is bounded by limitations of vision as stated by Legge, Cheung, Yu, Chung, Lee, and Owens (2007). Further, Huestegge, Radach, Corbie, and Huestegge (2009) reported that second graders, on the average, made saccadic excursions of 5.27 letter spaces, whereas fourth graders made a saccadic movement that traversed 6.32 letter spaces. McConkie and Zola (1989) reported that college students average saccadic excursions of 7.2 letter spaces.

After vision recovers, orthographic identification of letters begins and the word being fixated upon is decoded, or recognized, automatically. Then there is a shift of attention to the right peripheral area as a guide to where to move; vision drops, and then readers prepare to make a move to the next fixation.

Words fed into short-term memory are first stored as letter configurations, hopefully instantly recognized as words. Then after one, two, or more fixations, recognition is confirmed as words are fused into phrases and later realized in terms of meaning. Kliegl, Nuthmann, and Engbert (2006) depicted this process as "eye-movement lag."

The majority of people are unaware of the number of fixations they make in relation to the number of words they have read. The average adult reading a 10-word line will tend to make from eight to 10 fixations. A superior reader will make perhaps five fixations, while a child in elementary school will fixate from 13 to 22 times. An individual referred to as a "word-by-word" reader does not make just one eye stop per word, but usually makes two or more fixations per word. We are not aware of this amount of visual activity, because of the subtlety of the activity involved and our lack of direct, conscious control.

McConkie and Rayner (1976) stated, "There is guidance during reading on the basis of peripheral visual patterns." Hoffman and Subramaniam (1995) also provided evidence that the viso-spacial attention is required to execute a saccade. Rayner and Morrison (1981) and others refer to this process as parafovial preprocessing. Posner (1980) stated, "It is possible to move attention without moving our eyes."

Thus beyond the area of print that can be perceived with reasonable acuity, the print in the right periphery can furnish information as to where the next fixation might land.

It is a well-established fact that more efficient readers require fewer fixations to read a given line of text than poorer readers. This fact is cited in the Report of the National Reading Panel (2000), which also found that in a national study of fourth graders, 44 percent of the students were found to be disfluent. This panel concludes that children who do not develop reading fluency, no matter how bright they are, will continue to read slowly.

Further, a reader who is maturing, in terms of reading efficiency, tends to reduce the number of fixations. Certainly it is desirable to acquire visual/functional and perceptual habits and cognitive competence that result in a minimum amount of ocular activity, for, generally, the greater the number of fixations, the more time spent reading, and the more energy consumed in the reading process. An individual might employ a comparatively large number of fixations for any of the following reasons:

Difficulty with Visual Acuity or Binocular Coordination

Any inability to see with good visual acuity or to coordinate the eyes properly will tend to increase the number of fixations, as well as regressions, especially those corrective regressions (reverse direction fixations) occurring in the beginning of each new line of print.

Conditioning of Early Reading Experiences

As mentioned previously, an excessive number of fixations and regressions can become part of an individual's habitual oculomotor performance due to the conditioning that occurs during the early stages of learning to read, in which a considerable number of new words are introduced weekly. Also possible is an overstress on phonics, in which the amount of time needed to consciously analyze letters and letter sounds delays the silent reading process.

All of these early learning experiences can contribute to the formation of an inefficient oculomotor activity, or a less-than-fluent approach to silent reading, and often become rather habitual by the intermediate grades.

Perceptual Factors

The manner in which an individual perceives words, discriminates, and recognizes words accurately and retains them (visual memory) influences the manner in which the reader will perform during silent reading. If the learned reading behavior of the subject is to overscrutinize visual material and to "double check" excessively, this perceptual requirement will typically condition the use of an excess number of fixations and regressions.

Comprehension Difficulties

If the comprehension ability of a subject is poor, the tendency will be for that reader to employ an excess number of fixations, as he or she pauses and ponders, attempting to achieve understanding.

Determining the Number of Fixations

The Visagraph automatically calculates the number of fixations employed by a subject reading 100 words as shown in the following table.

Table 4.2

Taylor National Norms																		
	Grade Level													Advanced				
	1	2	3	4	5	6	7	8	9	10	11	12	Col.	1	2	3	4	5
Fixations/100 Words	224	174	155	139	129	120	114	109	105	101	96	94	90	77	65	57	48	44

"Grade Level Norms for the Components of the Fundamental Reading Skill," by Stanford E. Taylor, Helen Frackenpohl, and James L. Pettee, EDL Research and Information Bulletin No. 3, Educational Developmental Laboratories, Inc., 1960.
Advanced—Represents typical reading performance characteristics for trained readers.

Nature of Regressions

Regressions are reverse fixations and are those fixations that occur following a right-to-left saccade. Many of the causes for regressions have been discussed in the section on fixations as stemming from less-than-satisfactory visual acuity or binocular coordination problems, conditioning during "beginning-to-read" stages, perceptual inadequacies, and poor or unsatisfactory comprehension. However, regressions can be classified into three types: those that are habitual, those that are caused by reading difficulties of the moment, and others that are seemingly neurologically activated.

Habitual regressions typically result from inadequate formation of an effective directional attack when learning to read. As a consequence, some students incorporate or employ a certain amount of corrective movement in reading each line of print. This habit can become so ingrained that regressions will occur at similar points in every line of print.

Other individuals may incorporate a number of regressions into their reading performance by virtue of a lack of reading confidence and an ingrained need to "double check" words and context. Their general insecurity, in terms of remembering what they have read, is sufficiently great to cause them to regress and even reread habitually.

If a person's second fixation on making a return sweep to a new line of print is a regression, this is usually caused by lack of proper coordination between the vergence of the two eyes, permitting single vision. This condition occurs most commonly with a hyperopic (far-sighted) person, who, during the return sweep, tries to adjust vergence and focus to permit single, clear vision, and in doing so, characteristically overconverges and overaccommodates. The result is inaccuracy in executing a full return sweep and print that is not clear.

Consequently, the hyperopic person will employ a corrective or regressive fixation on each new line of print, to relocate more accurately on the new line of print and perceive more clearly, as cited by Taylor (1937 & 1966) and shown in Figure 4.4. This type of regressive fixation is not counted as a regression, for it is a portion of the return sweep activity.

Sporadic regressions result principally from difficulty with the content. Perceptual errors, inadequate interpretive or organizational ability, and/or lack of experience create the need to check back. Whether

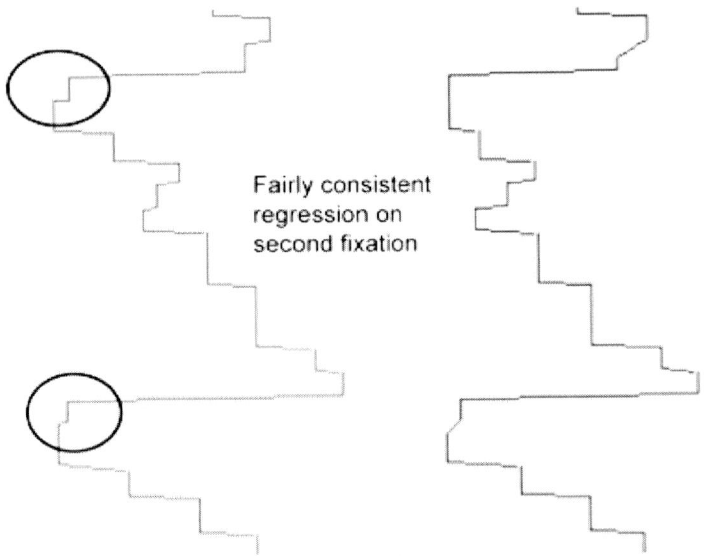

Figure 4.4

such regressions actually accomplish a "second look," or whether they are rather instinctive momentary pause reactions stemming from a subconscious awareness of mental confusion, has not been clearly established. In this regard, it should also be noted that regressions may not occur at the instant of perceptual confusion, but be delayed in time.

Clusters occur in individuals who will, at intervals, exhibit a cluster of regressions. Cluster regressions are two or more regressions in succession at different points in reading, for no apparent reason, based on content, vision, etc. Pavlidis and Miles (1981) associate this occurrence with a condition of dyslexia. They cite, as additional symptoms, excessively large saccades in conjunction with such regressions. This type of occurrence, however, needs further study.

It is important to note that, while a small percentage of regressive movements may be a reflection of the immediate situation or influenced by conscious control, the majority of regressions seem habitual. As previously mentioned, the studies by Carmichael and Dearborn (1947); Seibert (1943); and Taylor, Frackenpohl, and Pettee (1959) indicate that the number of regressions a reader makes is as consistent as the number of his or her total fixations.

Regressions require only fractions of a second (perhaps only .24 seconds), and because they are interspersed with forward fixations, the reader is seldom conscious of their occurrence. Although the time required for a single regression is small, total time spent in regressions might occupy from one-fifth to one-third of the total reading time. Desirably the proportion of regressions to total fixations should not exceed 10 to 15 percent. Again Pavlidis and Miles (1981) cite some dyslexic readers as averaging as much as 30 to 80 percent of these fixations as regressive movements.

It is important to distinguish between regressing and the more conscious act of rereading (in which cases there will usually be extra lines read). Regressions occur after small reverse direction interfixation movements, singly or several in sequence. While sometimes considered as regressing (true only when the person rereads on the same line), rereading usually refers to returning to a previously read section of a line of print, or sentences, paragraphs, or pages. Rereading is usually caused by lack of confidence, poor comprehension, or lack of attention. It is productive only in study-type reading activities, such as text reading, content analysis, literary appreciation, etc. Rereading is most typically identified by large saccades (much longer than interfixation movements), followed by the rereading of sections of lines or entire lines that have been previously read.

As the Taylor Norm Report (1960) shows in Table 4.3, students in the earlier grades will average a greater number of regressions than students in the intermediate grades or higher.

Table 4.3

Taylor National Norms																		
	Grade Level													Advanced				
	1	2	3	4	5	6	7	8	9	10	11	12	Col.	1	2	3	4	5
Regressions/100 Words	52	40	35	31	28	25	23	21	20	19	18	17	15	11	8	5	4	2

"Grade Level Norms for the Components of the Fundamental Reading Skill," by Stanford E. Taylor, Helen Frackenpohl, and James L. Pettee, EDL Research and Information Belletin No. 3, Educational Developmental Laboratories, Inc., 1960.
Advanced—Represents typical reading-performance characteristics for trained readers.

Nature of Average Span of Recognition

The span of recognition refers to the number of words or word parts perceived during a fixation or eye pause during reading. Span of recognition does not refer to the amount of print material impinging on the retina of the eye, but rather to the number of words a reader recognizes or can deal with interpretively. In reading, "perceptions" are so interrelated that it is unrealistic to think of span of recognition as a measurement during an isolated seeing situation. When considering a person's span of recognition during reading, we must look to a reader's performance throughout the reading of a selection as providing a more typical reflection of his or her average visual intake of words or word parts, as shown in Figure 4.5.

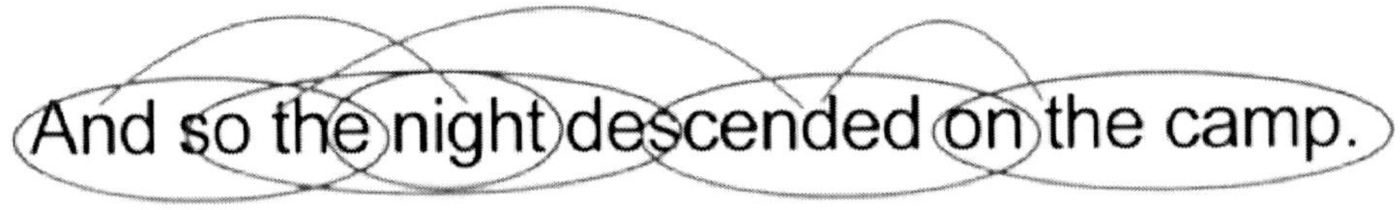

Figure 4.5

As stated by Carmichael and Dearborn (1947), "It is difficult to answer the question of how much a reader apprehends during a fixation pause, if only because it is extremely likely that more had been seen than can be reported. Cues from the print on either side of the fixation point may have been grasped, which, though they are not reportable, are useful in the perception of what has been read during the fixation pause or of what will be read during the next fixation pause. Peripheral vision may also aid in the determination of where the next fixation pause is to be located."

Research continues regarding the size of the span of recognition and the various influences of print and context on span of recognition, and undoubtedly will continue in the future. However, the calculation we refer to as average span of recognition (determined by noting the number of fixations required to read the designated 100 words) in the Visagraph recording is the most significant measure when judging a reader's performance efficiency.

The Visagraph recording computes the average span of recognition, fully realizing that there is undoubtedly some variation in span of recognition from fixation to fixation, and that some words may have been "skipped." And although it is possible with the Visagraph to detect the approximate number of letters traversed in interfixation movements, one cannot directly relate this letter information to what was actually perceived (cognitively) during each fixation.

However, judging from the usual reading patterns of most readers, this variation of perceptual span would not seem to be extreme. Most readers above grade four tend to maintain their characteristic number of fixations per line throughout a selection in relation to the words per line. Notably, within any given line, they do not fluctuate significantly in the extent of saccadic movement.

Perhaps more misconceptions have arisen about the span of recognition than about any other aspect of the reading activity. In any number of textbooks, articles, and manuals, references have been made to the ability of children to "see" in phrases during reading and to the ability of adults to "take in at a glance" four or five words, sentences, and even paragraphs. This misconception can be traced in part to tachistoscopic theories and techniques, which propose that persons can be trained to "see" four and five word phrases at 1/100 of a second. It is important to realize, however, that the seeing accomplished during tachistoscopic exposures differs greatly from that taking place during reading.

During tachistoscopic exposures, an individual's level of attention is considerably higher than is typical of continuous reading. Further, the "seeing" that is accomplished during a tachistoscopic exposure is not followed by other perceptions, which have the effect of reducing span of recognition in continuous reading, as substantiated by Gilbert (1959b). Nor is there the usual kinesthesia of continuous movements, as in reading, which further reduces span of recognition, as indicated by Gilbert (1959a).

In a pilot study with an eye-movement camera carried out by this author, it was shown that the span of a person involved in tachistoscopic exercises was considerably larger than his or her span when reading material of the same level of difficulty. For instance, one subject showed that he could easily perceive four- to five-word phrases during a tachistoscopic exposure of 1/100 of a second, while in continuous reading he showed an average span of recognition of only 1.6 words.

As you can see from Table 4.4, a first grader at the end of the year perceives an average of only .45 of a word per eye stop; students do not average a full word until eleventh grade; and even the average college student only 1.11 words, reading at the rate of 280 words per minute. Even after tachistoscopic and reading instrument training, the span for an excellent reader seldom exceeds 2.5 words.

Table 4.4

Taylor National Norms																		
	Grade Level													Advanced				
	1	2	3	4	5	6	7	8	9	10	11	12	Col.	1	2	3	4	5
Average Span of Recognition	.45	.57	.65	.72	.78	.83	.88	.92	.95	.99	1.04	1.06	1.11	1.30	1.53	1.75	2.08	2.27

"Grade Level Norms for the Components of the Fundamental Reading Skill," by Stanford E. Taylor, Helen Frackenpohl, and James L. Pettee, EDL Research and Information Belletin No. 3, Educational Developmental Laboratories, Inc., 1960.
Advanced—Represents typical reading performance characteristics for trained readers.

Further substantiation for the small amount perceived per eye stop during reading is contained in a study by Gray (1956), conducted at the University of Chicago, where eye-movement recordings were made of adults from 14 different countries reading their native languages. The average silent reading span was only 1.6 words, which is what one would expect for people who are mature and undoubtedly advanced readers.

Eye-movement recording studies by McConkie and Rayner (1976) have further determined the extent of a reader's span of recognition, as shown in Figure 4.6. College students were recorded in reading situations in which letters in words were altered at various letter positions to the left and to the right of a reader's fixation position to determine the extent of sensitivity of a reader's span. McConkie and Rayner determined that the college-level reader was sensitive to only four letters to the left and six to eight letters to the right of the fixation point, equivalent in total to two words or fewer.

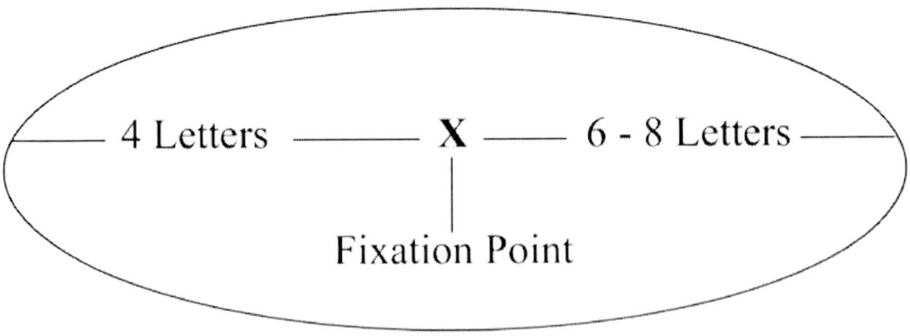

Figure 4.6

Studies by Legge et al. (2007) describe the limitations of visual span as being determined by limitations of vision; in essence, the explorations they set forth preclude expectations of phrase perception during reading.

Earlier studies by Feinberg (1949) determined that seven to eight letter spaces away from the fixation point is where visual acuity drops to approximately 45 percent and then rapidly diminishes beyond that distance. This reduction in acuity is reflected in Figure 4.7 by the author, and it is in line with the findings of Feinberg (1949), Legge et al. (2007), and McConkie and Rayner (1976).

It is apparent, then, that phrase seeing during reading is a myth. Realizing, however, that all readers, even beginners in first grade, "think" in phrases and larger linguistic units, we can only conclude

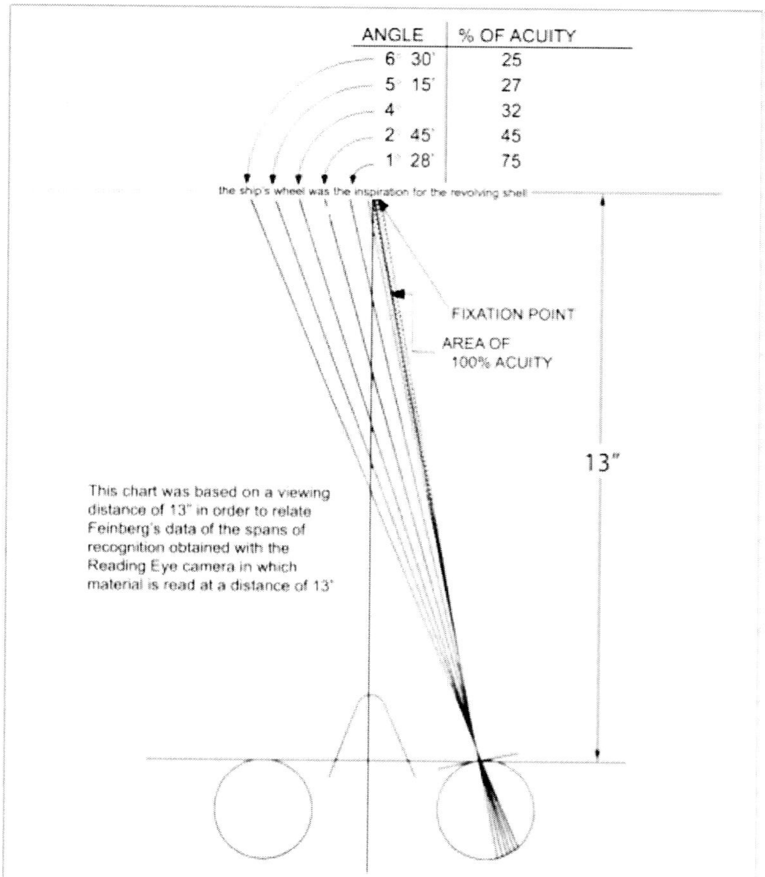

Figure 4.7

that a person constructs a thought through a series of fixations in which a series of visual impressions are processed in short-term memory.

Nature of Average Duration of Fixation

The duration of fixation refers to the length of time a reader's eyes typically pause during fixations. In eye-movement recording, we use the term "average duration of fixation," which is computed from the overall time (in seconds) it takes a reader to read a selection and the total number of fixations employed to read the selection.

It should be noted that in past eye-movement recording computations, the length of time required for the interfixation movements and return sweeps was included as part of the fixation time or reading time; consequently, the average duration of fixation included time for saccadic movement. This does not detract from the usefulness of the final calculation of average duration of fixation, since the saccadic movement occupies such a slight amount of time, approximately only .15 seconds for a word or seven letters, according to Rayner, Pollatsek, Ashby, and Clifton, Jr. (2012), and does not shorten significantly with maturation.

In the Visagraph, beyond the average duration of fixation calculations, the actual duration of each fixation is also presented in the Model Graph with Values. This would show the actual time spent in each fixation.

As you can see from Table 4.5, an elementary school child might pause as long as .33 seconds per eye stop, making about three movements per second. (This is undoubtedly influenced by the fact that the student's reading experience is predominantly oral, and the fact that he or she does not recognize a great many words easily and quickly, and thus does not associate very rapidly.) A more mature reader might average .24 seconds per eye stop, making slightly more than four fixations per second. The shortest duration found in thousands of eye-movement photographs of reading was .16 seconds or six fixations per second, but it should be noted that this reader, although a rapid reader, was not extraordinarily rapid, for the exceptionally short duration was offset by a greater number of fixations and a correspondingly small average span of recognition.

Table 4.5

Taylor National Norms																		
	Grade Level													Advanced				
Average Duration of Fixation (seconds)	1	2	3	4	5	6	7	8	9	10	11	12	Col.	1	2	3	4	5
	.33	.30	.28	.27	.27	.27	.27	.27	.27	.26	.26	.25	.24	.23	.23	.22	.22	.22

"Grade Level Norms for the Components of the Fundamental Reading Skill," by Stanford E. Taylor, Helen Frackenpohl, and James L. Pettee, EDL Research and Information Bulletin No. 3, Educational Developmental Laboratories, Inc., 1960.
Advanced—Represents typical reading performance characteristics for trained readers.

In general, duration of fixation tends to shorten as the reader matures, reflecting a decrease in reaction time and an increase in the rapidity with which the reader associates and comprehends. However, as you will note from the Average Duration of Fixation Table, duration changes but little after a child reaches fourth grade or 10 to 11 years of age.

Most probably the reason for the small amount of change from fourth grade on lies in the fact that the reader's organizational, perceptual, and visual/functional maturation reflects itself principally in a reduction of fixations and regressions and an increase in span of recognition. The fact that more visual material must now be dealt with per fixation undoubtedly contributes to the small change in duration. Thus there would appear to be a balance or personal equation in each reader in terms of the number of fixations (reflected in span of recognition) and the average duration of fixation.

That this might be the case is evidenced further by the results of reading improvement courses in which people have developed considerable fluency in reading or reading efficiency (reflected in a pronounced reduction of fixations and regressions and a corresponding improvement in rate), yet the duration has changed but slightly. As a rule, the duration of fixation does shorten, particularly if a reader's duration was longer than .24 seconds before training. Sometimes average duration of fixation will remain the same, and in other cases, increase slightly. These conditions occur predominantly when the reader's duration of fixation before training was shorter than .23 seconds. In the situations where a person's duration remains the same or is lengthened slightly after training, the overall reading time was reduced as well as the number of fixations employed to perceive the material. Thus it is probable that a reader required the same duration interval (or longer) to "see" and "process" more per fixation.

It should be mentioned that today, in many eye-movement research studies, the term "gaze duration" is mentioned. Gaze duration is a sum total of all of the fixations and regressions spent on a given word during reading. This term, although meaningful in specific research studies, does not apply in the Visagraph analysis in which the overall number of fixations is reported in relation to total reading time.

Reading Rate with Comprehension

The term "rate" refers to the time required by a reader to read through a particular selection while displaying comprehension. Probably no term in reading has more interpretations than the term "rate of reading."

A measurement of rate of words per minute has the most validity when it refers to a usual manner of reading, or the way the person might typically read a magazine, novel, or other non-test situations, where rereading or reflection are at a minimal level. It is more meaningful to refer to a person's "usual" rate as a rate at which narrative informational material is read, rather than a skimming rate where only portions of the context are read, or a slower rate for reflective or analytical reading, which requires pauses to reflect and perhaps visualize. A person's usual rate is the rate designation referred to in Visagraph recordings.

It is interesting to note that Carver (1989) documents the fact that the Taylor rate norms reflect the performance of students in various grade levels when test selections were read with 70 percent or higher comprehension. Besides being an unusually large national sample (12,143 students in grades one through college level), the Taylor data has the advantage of reflecting the comprehension rates reported by Carver on the Nelson Denny test, as well as the Neuropathy, Ataxia, and Retinitis Pigmentosa (NARP) data.

While rate cannot be meaningfully considered apart from comprehension, there are certain factors that greatly influence the relative rapidity with which a reader moves through print. Among these will be a reader's binocular coordination competence, his or her perceptual accuracy and efficiency, and the oculomotor activity, which has become habitual over the years. These factors prevent rate from being directly proportional to the difficulty of the content, or to the experiences of the reader, or to the comprehension achieved. In other words, many people, particularly poorer or less-efficient readers, will not vary greatly in their reading rate on different levels of material, unless the difficulty of the material becomes overwhelming. Some readers' comprehension will be poor no matter how slowly they read. And there are readers whose comprehension improves as they consciously attempt to increase their rate, and others who exhibit lower comprehension as they exert conscious effort to increase their rate.

Many people assume that rate is a highly variable factor and that we can, at will, alter our rate to suit the situation of our purposes. In actuality, the vast majority of people vary their rate only slightly on material that could be classified as easy to fairly difficult. They may, upon encountering reflective or analytical reading material, slow down due to the perceptual, interpretive, and associative complexities inherent in the material. These people usually do not accelerate their reading on easy or light material because to do so would require a greater outlay of energy. Rather, the majority maintains, with a somewhat limited range, a performance rate that is comfortable and reasonably effective. The studies of Ballantine (1951); Morse (1951); and Taylor, Frackenpohl, and Pettee (1959) involving changes in the difficulty of material, and the study of Seibert (1943) involving changes in subject matter, all support the proposition that people tend to maintain the same performance rate over a wide range of content.

The ability to vary one's rate for various types of reading material would seem to be a desirable capability, but unfortunately, it is possible for only the most efficient readers, those who have sufficient visual/functional, perceptual capability, and interpretive flexibility to allow them to perform comfortably and efficiently at various rates. This was further borne out by another eye-movement photography study by Taylor, Frackenpohl, and Pettee (1959) in which eighth graders were first photographed reading in their usual manner, then instructed to read with the same degree of comprehension, but faster, for a reward. In this study, the students were able to increase their rate somewhat, but not without significant loss of comprehension. This further emphasizes a person's reliance on a characteristic manner of reading when comprehension is the goal.

It should be noted that, in many cases, readers will seemingly effect an increase or decrease in rate by altering their strategies and organizational approach to reading content: survey a chapter, note headings, sub-headings, marginal notes, and so on, or employ a "skimming" approach, looking purposefully for certain ideas or information. This is not to say that the reader is necessarily reading faster, for it would be inaccurate to say that the passing over of words or pages was truly reading. Rather the person is altering his or her interpretive emphasis toward "looking," locating, and then reading.

Grayum's (1953) study of skimming offers further reinforcement regarding the above. In this study, fourth graders through adult readers were given selections of light reading material. Eye-movement records of these people were taken, and from them the author noted: "Techniques observed in skimming included skipping words in various degrees, marked changed in rate, pausing, regressing, looking back, and looking ahead." In those parts of the selections read most thoroughly, the person appeared to employ a usual manner of reading.

Grayum notes, "In that part of the selection read most slowly, every line was covered by two or three fixations per line, while in the part read most rapidly, there were five sweeps across the card of 12 lines, with one or two fixations per 'line' across the card as shown by the photographs." The overall average of words per fixation was 2.65 for the better skimmers. Allowing for the lines and words skipped, the span and performance on the sections read thoroughly was very close to that usually characteristic of the reader.

Consider also that the reading performance of so many people is characterized by rereading, or "looking back" over material already read. The usual rate (as measured by eye-movement recording) may be obscured by this type of performance on a standardized test. In general the majority of people appear to read slightly faster during eye-movement recording than they do on a standardized test (stemming from the fact that they are asked to read the selection one time and to avoid rereading). This is not to say that the rate measured by a standardized test is not valid, but rather to indicate that the factor of rereading is not included in the measurement of rate of reading on such tests.

Many claims are made regarding the high rates at which certain people can read. It is not uncommon to hear rates of 1,000 to 6,000 words per minute discussed as being within the reach of the average person in speed-reading courses. Seemingly, there is no evidence to substantiate these statements. There are undoubtedly a few exceptional readers who attain fairly phenomenal rates, but the performance of these people should not be confused with what is possible for the average person.

As we mentioned previously, it is important to differentiate between truly rapid reading and skimming. As stated by Gilbert (1956), "People who are credited with such feats are actually engaging in a highly proficient type of scanning or skimming. Unquestionably, masterful skimming is an extremely valuable study skill, but it is not to be confused with thorough reading."

This author (1962) analyzed the oculomotor performance of a number of Air Academy Kadets through eye-movement recording, as these students were engaged in the Evelyn Woods speed reading program, and found that almost all the Kadets reading at rates above 600 words per minute were actually employing a skimming process as they moved down the center of the columns of print, and were not involved in a continuous thorough reading. Their comprehension was only 50 percent or less using the skimming approach, whereas their comprehension was 90 percent or greater when they read in a conventional manner.

The rate of reading as applied to the Visagraph eye-movement recording is based on the following conditions:

- The level of test material read is such that it permits a reasonable degree of fluency to be demonstrated.
- Comprehension is adequate (70 percent or better).
- The test selections are structured so that they are reasonably complete in themselves, with their facts and ideas presented in a sequential manner.

During the eye-movement reading process, a subject may be told to read as rapidly as possible, but primarily cautioned to read for comprehension. (Following every test, questions are asked to judge whether or not the student read to the best of his or her ability.)

Table 4.6 provides an indication of the average rate demonstrated by students at various levels when reading material at their grade level. In addition the average adult has been found to read at rates ranging from 175 to 300 words per minute, with an average rate of 225 words per minute. The superior adult reader might average 500 words per minute and even the best readers, after completing a reading

Table 4.6

Taylor National Norms																		
	Grade Level													Advanced				
WPM Rate with Comprehension	1	2	3	4	5	6	7	8	9	10	11	12	Col.	1	2	3	4	5
	80	115	138	158	173	185	195	204	214	224	237	250	280	340	400	480	560	620

"Grade Level Norms for the Components of the Fundamental Reading Skill," by Stanford E. Taylor, Helen Frackenpohl, and James L. Pettee, EDL Research and Information Belletin No. 3, Educational Developmental Laboratories, Inc., 1960.
Advanced—Represents typical reading performance characteristics for trained readers.

improvement course, rarely read above rates of 650 words per minute. In general, there appears to be an upper rate-of-reading limit of 800 words per minute for even the most proficient and accomplished reader.

This condition results most likely from the very "restricted" span of recognition of most readers (seldom exceeding 2.5 words per fixation) in combination with the maximum number of eye movements that can be made per second (rarely over five per second). Multiplying these factors (and excluding the effect of any regressions) yields a reading rate of 750 words per minute. Consider also that individuals who do employ a large span of recognition usually average fewer fixations per second, most typically four.

Substantiation for this reduced span of recognition, by virtue of limitations of visual acuity, can be found in the research by Feinberg (1949), as well as Legge et al. (2007). Substantiation for the maximum number of fixations per second can be found in the research by Buswell (1935), Taylor (1960), and Volkmann (1962).

Reading Rate without Rereading

This is helpful information in comparing a subject's performance in pre- and post-tests where one Visagraph test might have involved rereading. This allows more equivalent comparison of reading performance efficiency over a period of time, typically before and after fluency development training.

The rate with comprehension includes any rereading. The rate adjusted for rereading is a calculation that eliminates any effect of rereading. Any intraline rereading (instances in which a regressive movement is greater than 30 percent of the line value, which typically exceeds usual regressive activity) and any extra lines read by a student are deleted by extrapolation in this calculation.

Directional Attack Difficulty

The term "directional attack" refers to the tendency of the reader to perceive and organize content in a sequential left-to-right manner. The perceptual activity and the visual patterns in reading are so interrelated that it may be said that the recorded pattern indicates, in a general manner, both the perceptual accuracy of the individual and his or her orderliness in dealing with the content. Thus the oculomotor pattern made by the reader's eyes reveals the quality and nature of his or her directional attack and is as individualistic as are the components themselves.

The quality of a reader's directional attack relates directly to the manner in which words are fed into short-term memory. When the sequence of visual impressions is rapid, sequential, and regular, it can be assumed that the word impressions being processed in short-term memory are likewise sequential and reinforcing syntactically as a result. Likewise, poor directional attack would suggest a more imperfect non-syntactical and less reinforcing, wandering, input into short-term memory, which will require cognitive organization to "straighten out" the message.

The Visagraph automatically reports Directional Attack Difficulty as a calculation of the percentage of regressions to total fixations. Generally, should the percentage of regressions be 10 to 15 percent or less, a reader's directional attack can be judged relatively efficient. If the percentage is 25 percent or more, the reader is employing a less than desirable directional attack. (There have been many instances in which the percentage of regressions has been as high as 40 percent or more.) The exception to these percentages lies with superior readers, reading at rates of 600 words per minute or more, who might have a residue of a few regressions, which, when compared with a relatively small number of fixations, might yield a high percentage. With such readers this percentage would not be significant.

Grade Level Efficiency

The Visagraph will automatically calculate a reader's overall reading efficiency and equivalent Grade Level Efficiency (GLE) performance.

"Relative Efficiency" is a calculation that provides an objective numerical indication of the grade level equivalent of a subject's reading performance. This is based on the following considerations:

- It presupposes that fixations, regressions, and rate are the most important components (span and duration being calculations derived from these).
- It presupposes that a person who makes more regressions is generally less effective perceptually, and that regressions, therefore, should be given additional weight in the calculations (they are already included in the total count of fixations). See Figure 4.8.

$$\text{Relative Efficiency} = \frac{\text{Rate (wpm)}}{\text{Fixations per 100 words} + \text{Regressions per 100 Words}}$$

Figure 4.8

The number thus obtained can be considered the Relative Efficiency (RE) of the individual reading material on a given grade level. This RE can be compared with grade level averages by consulting Table 4.7, which is based on the norm study by S. E. Taylor, et al. (1960), in relation to fixations, regressions, and reading rate per grade level.

NOTE: Grade Level Efficiency derived from the Relative Efficiency Formula is a convenient and reliable indication of recording performance efficiency. There are instances where one might also look at the number of fixations and regressions, in relation to Grade and Goal calculations, for additional perspective to changes that result from reading fluency development programs.

Cross Correlation

Although the Cross Correlation report is designed to evaluate adequacy of binocular coordination, a very low cross correlation (perhaps .75 or lower) may signify the need for another recording. A poor recording can cause a low cross correlation. One can confirm the adequacy of a recording by comparing the Original Graph with the Model

Table 4.7

Relative Efficiency	Grade Level
.29	1.0
.41	1.5
.54	2.0
.63	2.5
.73	3.0
.83	3.5
.93	4.0
1.01	4.5
1.10	5.0
1.18	5.5
1.28	6.0
1.34	6.5
1.42	7.0
1.50	7.5
1.57	8.0
1.64	8.5
1.71	9.0
1.79	9.5
1.87	10.0
1.97	10.5
2.07	11.0
2.16	11.5
2.25	12.0
2.40	12.5
2.66	13.0
2.77	13.5
3.86	14.0 (Advanced 1)
5.48	15.0 (Advanced 2)
7.74	16.0 (Advanced 3)
10.77	17.0 (Advanced 4)
13.48	18.0 (Advanced 5)

Graph. If they seem very similar, the recording is probably satisfactory and the cross correlation is probably low because of coordination difficulties.

Generally, a cross correlation of less than 90 percent is cause for concern. There is usually some minor discrepancy in the movement (extent) of the amplitude of the two eyes that is not significant. Heller and Radach (1999) showed that variations in the amplitude between the two eyes could range between 1.0 and 1.5 letter spaces. A slight disparity of amplitude is undoubtedly compensated for by a reader's perceptual competence. Blythe, Liversedge, Joseph, White, Findlay, and Rayner (2006) reported that this disparity of a fixation and its variables are substantially greater for children. However, the College of Optometrists in Vision Development strongly suggests that in reading, a student must be able ". . . to aim the two eyes at the same point in terms of letter configurations to perceive letters clearly. Any difficulty with coordination can only result in visual discomfort as well as double or blurry word perception."

Grade Normative Performance

The profile plot, shown in Figure 4.9, displays a subject's reading performance characteristics in relation to Taylor's grade level norms.

Both of these plots extend to the left and right of a subject's Grade Level Efficiency determination. The lines on the chart to the left of a student's grade level show performance that is below grade level, whereas the lines to the right depict instances in which the student exceeds grade level expectations.

READING SIMULATION

Beyond the use of the Reading Report findings that may be discussed with students, there is a student's Simulation, shown in Figure 4.10, which displays exactly how a student read in terms of Fixations and Duration of Fixation. Presenting this Simulation to a student is tremendously motivating in terms of encouraging a student to want to improve his or her reading performance efficiency.

This display does not plot exact fixation locations, but does reason-

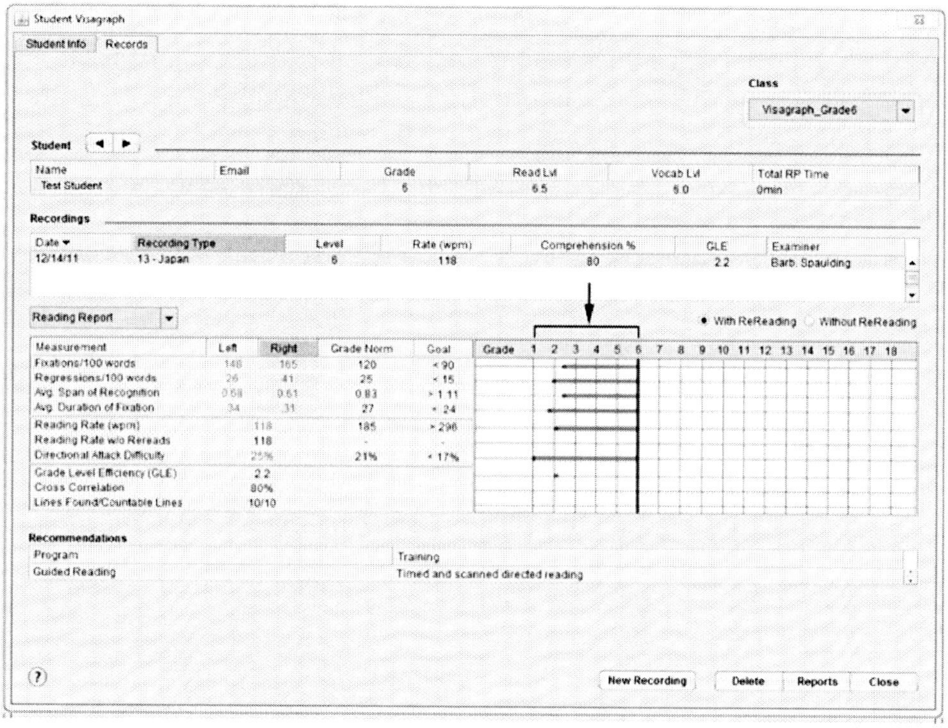

Figure 4.9

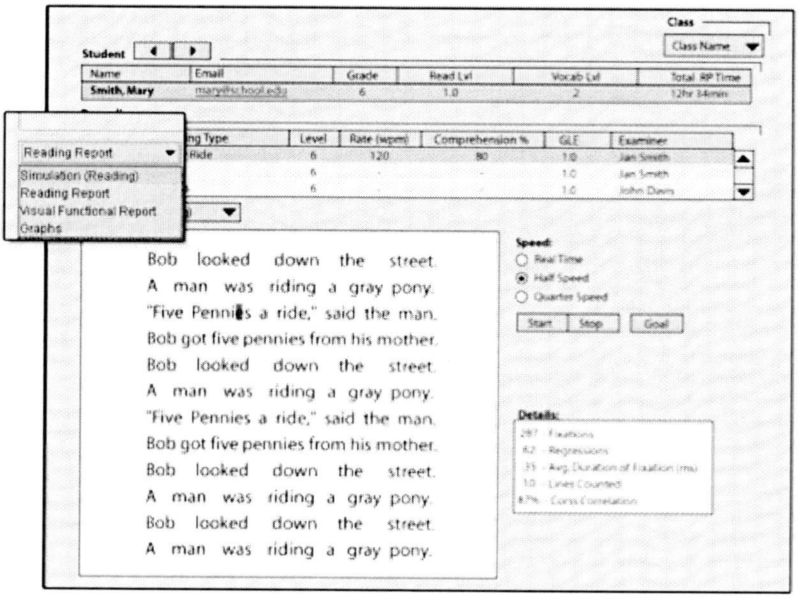

Figure 4.10

ably depict all fixations and regressions made on all lines displayed (beginning and ending lines excluded), as well as duration of fixation time. If the automatic analysis program could not detect all lines, the simulation will only display the number of lines detected starting with the second line of print and ending with the start of the last line (countable lines only).

Many students, when viewing the Simulation, respond positively to the fact that it is their poor reading skills that cause them difficulty in reading.

GRAPHS

In addition to the Reading and Visual/Functional data, there are two graphic displays of a student's visual and perceptual activity during reading–a Model Graph and an Original Graph.

Model Graph

The Model Graph, depicted in Figure 4.11, is a realigned plot that eliminates minor variations in visual performance to focus on the more meaningful performance characteristics that reflect a reader's Fundamental Reading Process. The display of the Model Graph shows the general factors analyzed.

Figure 4.12 points out information that is provided in a Model Graph.

To the left of the illustration is an indication of the ongoing total reading time in seconds. Following is a line-by-line notation that also indicates the number of each saccade indicating a new fixation on each line. The duration of each fixation is also displayed for the most active eye (used in the Reading Report). An examination of the consistency of a reader's performance throughout the reading of a selection is an indication of the level of maturity of the oculomotor activity.

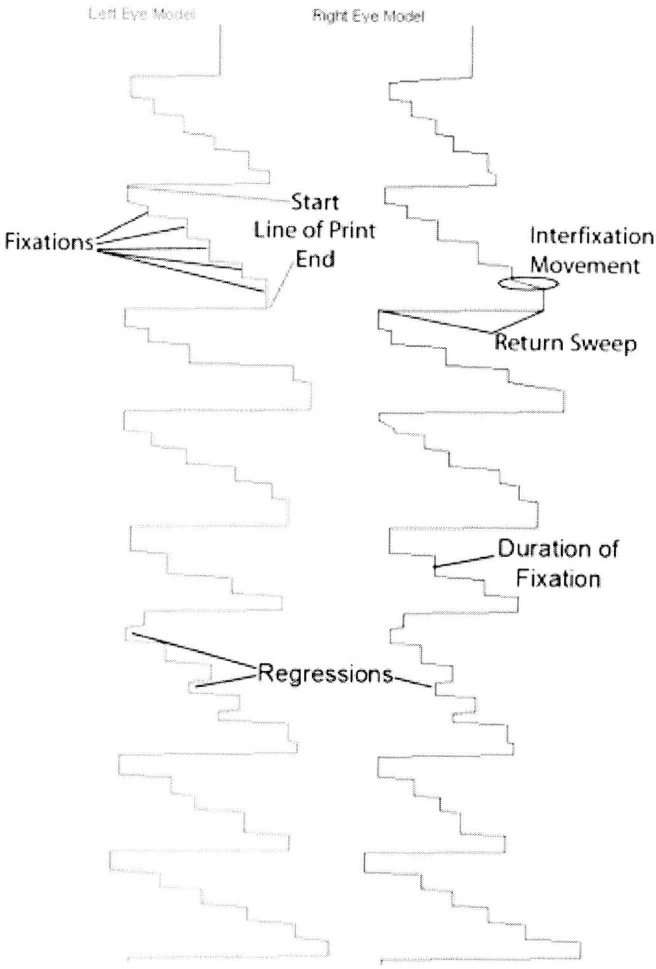
Left Eye Model
Right Eye Model
Start
Line of Print
End
Fixations
Interfixation
Movement
Return Sweep
Duration of
Fixation
Regressions

Figure 4.11

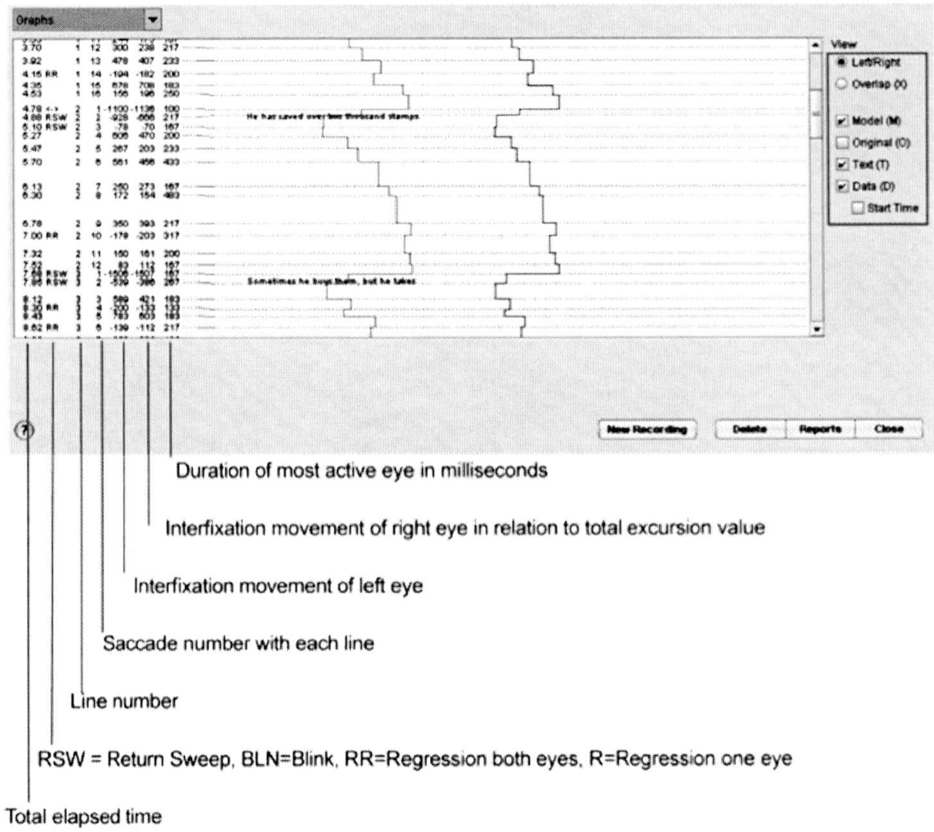

Figure 4.12

Original Graph

Figure 4.13 shows the Original Graph in which each movement of the eyes is minutely reported and is helpful in evaluating the points at which a student might have lost binocular control and experienced vergence problems.

Combination of Model Graph and Original Graph

If desired, both the Model Graph and the Original Graph can be displayed together, as shown in Figure 4.14, to gain further insights about binocular coordination.

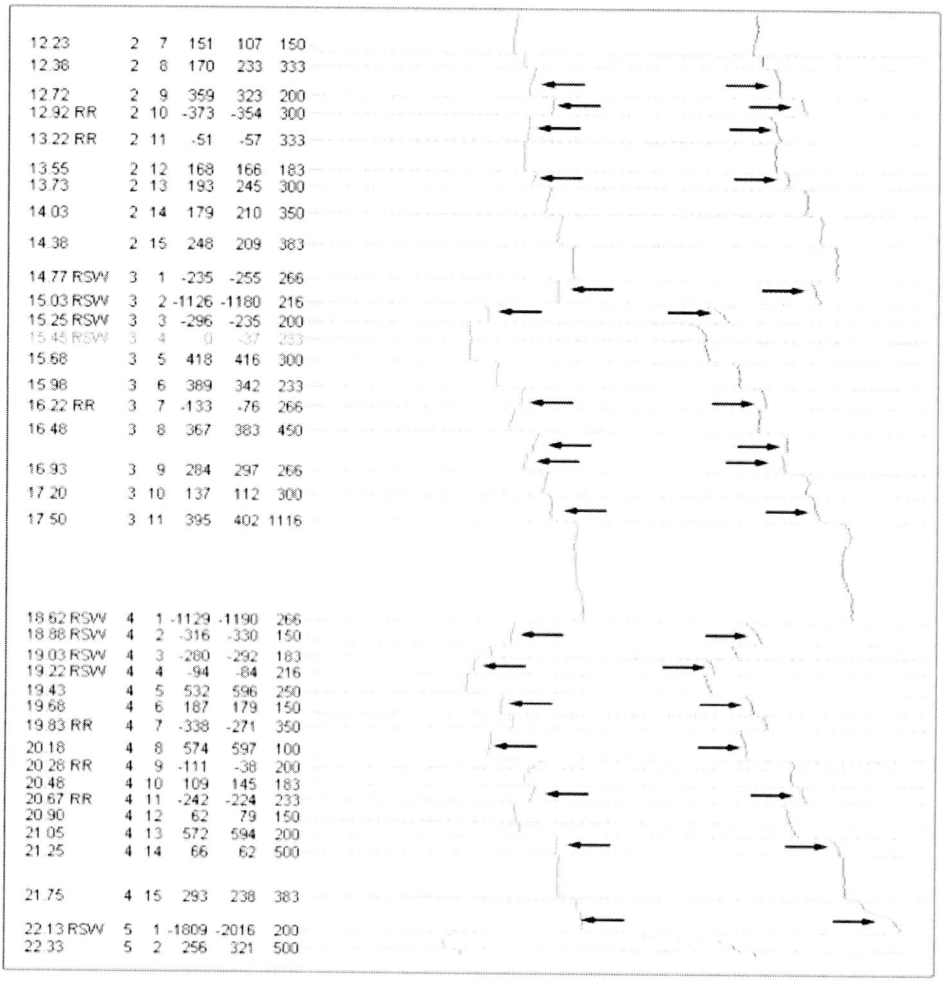

Figure 4.13

INTERPRETING THE VISUAL/FUNCTIONAL REPORT

Beyond the Reading Report, there is the Visual/Functional Report that reflects binocular coordination difficulties, as shown in Figure 4.15. This report, along with the responses to the Visagraph Student Inventory Questions, will indicate the severity of visual/functional ineffectiveness. This report is mostly of value to a reading specialist as opposed to a classroom teacher. Noting a low cross-correlation value in the Reading Report could require further exploration of a student's visual/functional limitations.

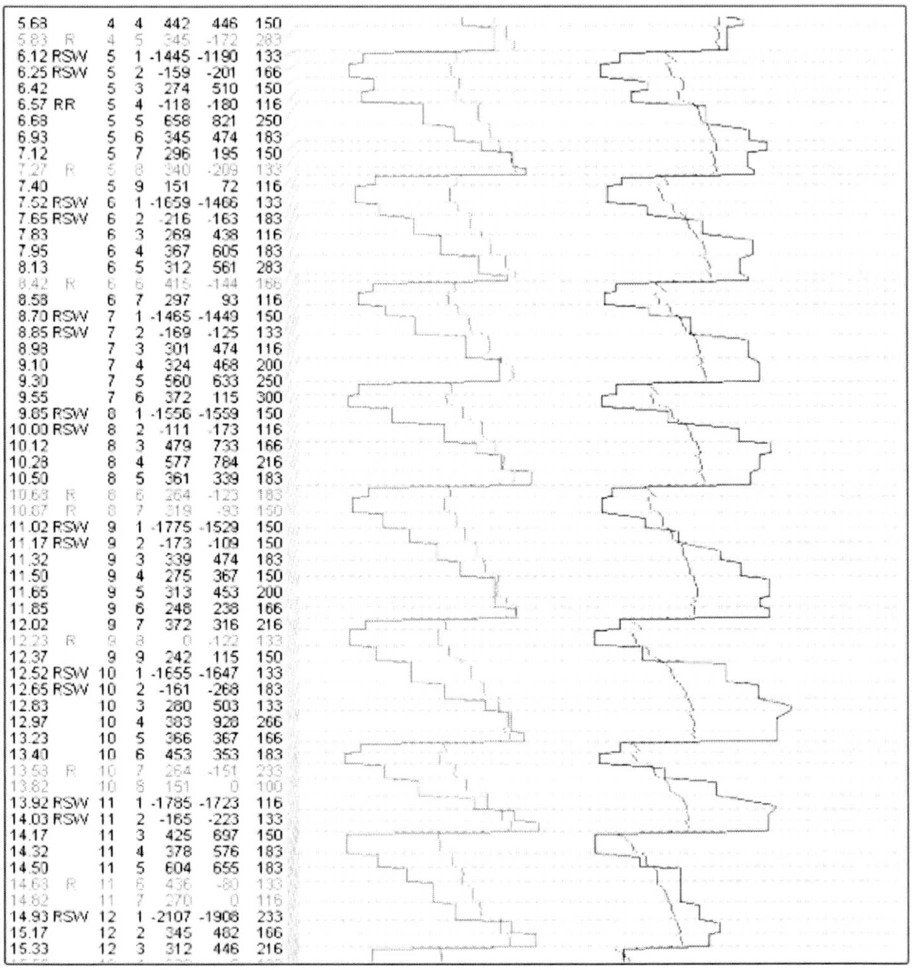

Figure 4.14

Fixations

In most instances, the performance of a subject's eyes will be quite similar. However instances where the difference in total fixations for both eyes exceeds 10 percent could be an indication of binocular coordination difficulty.

Regressions

A difference between the two eyes that exceeds 20 percent could also indicate difficulty with binocular coordination.

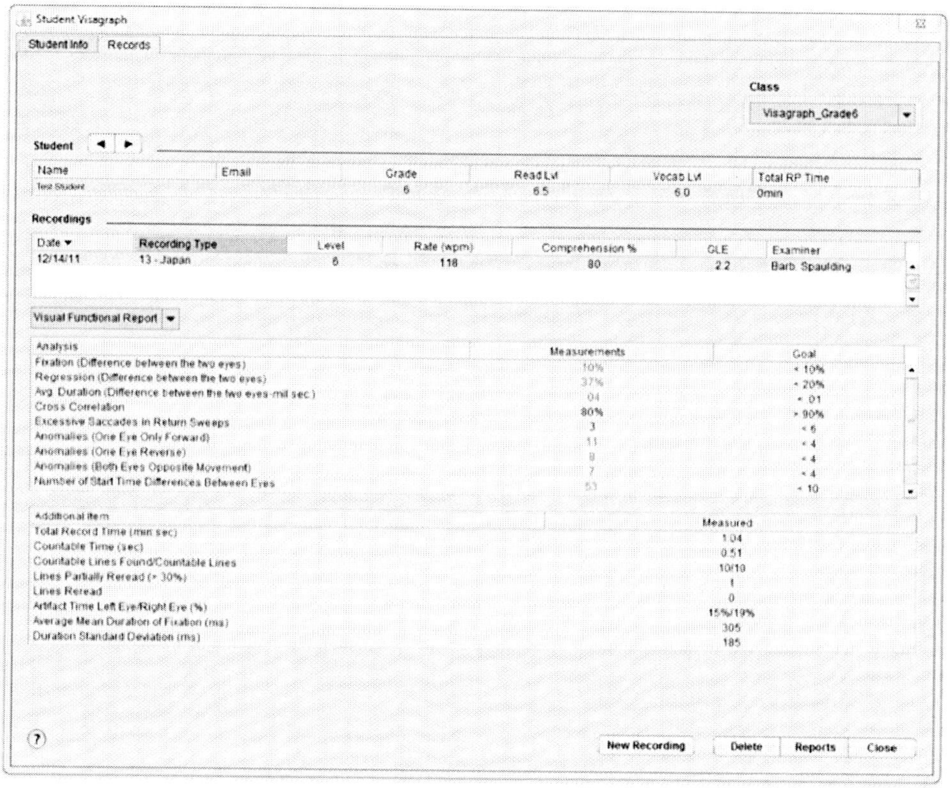

Figure 4.15

Average Duration (Difference Between the Two Eyes)

A difference of .01 between the two eyes could also be another indicator of binocular coordination difficulty.

Cross-Correlation

Cross-Correlation is an indicator of the degree to which the interfixational saccades of the two eyes are similar in excursion throughout the reading. A perfect correlation would be 1.000. Less than this would indicate some degree of difference in the similarity of saccades of the two eyes in either interfixation movement and/or return sweeps. Low correlations can be significant and should be studied. It is likely that a correlation less than .90 is suspect.

Excessive Saccades in Return Sweeps

Ideally, the number of return sweep saccades will equal the number of lines found. Any excess return sweep saccades indicate compensating movements made during the process of executing a return sweep. If a student's coordination or tracking is poor, the number of saccades and return sweeps can, at times, be two or perhaps three or more times the number of lines found. Return sweeps in excess of 50 percent or more of the total number of lines is another red flag that might indicate inadequate visual functioning.

Anomalies

Anomalies in excess of four in any of the three numbers reported can also signal visual/functional difficulty. These numbers reflect the following:

- The first number indicates instances in which one eye moved in a forward direction and the other eye did not move substantially enough to be recognized as a forward fixation. (The amount of movement to identify a movement as a new fixation is one percent of the total average line value. This is roughly equivalent to one or two letter spaces.)
- The second number indicates instances in which one eye moved in a reverse direction and the other eye did not move sufficiently to be detected as a new regressive fixation.
- The third number indicates the instances in which the two eyes appear to move in opposite directions. Whenever this occurs, it is best to examine the subject's original graph to be sure that the reported difference in the two eyes is truly significant. All anomalies will be presented in red in the values that can be employed in either the Model or Original graphs.

Start Time Differences Between Eyes

The nature of start time differences between the two eyes is counted and reported. To date, however, there are no criteria as to the number of start time differences that might support the consideration that this difference in start time reflects a coordination difficulty. An excessive number of such instances in conjunction with other reported data will simply add to an indication of visual/functional difficulty. You could compare the total number of fixations in relation to the start time differences in evaluating this data.

Student/Examiner Inventory

When a student's Visual Functional Report exhibits four or more indicators (in red) of possible visual impairments (low cross correlation, excessive return sweeps, anomalies, etc.), it is recommended that the Student Inventory Questions be administered and possibly the Teacher Inventory Questions as well.

These questions, which reflect a student's awareness of visual/functional problems, will often support the numerical findings revealed by the Visagraph. In instances where a parent or teacher's responses can be obtained, the examiner's questions are administered to further support an evaluation of a student's visual/functional difficulties. This information will then be added to the student's report. A student's or an examiner's responses to the questionnaire would likely validate the need for referral to a qualified vision specialist for a complete vision examination.

Obviously, the greater the number of adverse responses by a student or examiner, the greater the possibility that the student is experiencing visual/functional difficulty, and the greater likelihood of the need for referral.

Examiners may administer the Student Inventory Questions, as shown in Figure 4.16, from within the Student Visagraph panel on the Student Info tab.

The examiner may also complete a Teacher Inventory, as shown in Figure 4.17, based on observations of the subject.

After all 20 questions have been answered, the problematic responses will be displayed in red. Any responses to the questions that indicate inadequate adjustment to reading and/or near point activities can be a cause for concern. A total non-problematic/total questions will be listed with each completed inventory along with pertinent comments located beneath the inventory questions.

Reading Plus®

Visagraph® Student Inventory Questions

1. Do you like to read?
2. Do you get headaches when reading?
3. Can you read easily for 15 minutes?
4. Can you read easily for 30 minutes?
5. Can you read easily for 1 hour?
6. Can you read easily for 2 hours?
7. Do you get tired and sleepy when you read?
8. Do you study in short spurts?
9. Do your eyes get tired while reading?
10. Do your eyes get itchy while reading?
11. Do your eyes ever burn while reading?
12. Do your eyes get watery during reading?
13. Do the words in reading ever get muddy or blurred?
14. Do the letters in words double up or wiggle at times?
15. Do you find yourself saying the words to yourself during reading?
16. Do you have trouble understanding what you read?
17. Do you ever get car sick or headaches riding in a car?
18. Do you get a stiff neck or backache after reading?
19. Do you find your eyes bother you in sports such as baseball, basketball, tennis, or ping pong?
20. Do you feel your reading can be improved?

Figure 4.16

DETECTION OF VISUAL/FUNCTIONAL PROBLEMS

Suggestions for Referral to a Vision Specialist

There are five sources of data yielded by a Visagraph recording that might be studied in deciding whether a student should be referred to

Reading Plus®

Visagraph® Teacher Inventory Questions

1. Is student's level of academic achievement satisfactory for his/her age and/or grade?
2. Has progress been satisfactory in reading?
3. Has the student repeated any grade?
4. Is the student interested in school?
5. Does the student fatigue easily during reading and study tasks?
6. Is there a tendency to study in spurts?
7. Is there a tendency for the student to be easily distracted during reading?
8. Does the student seem to be happy and well adjusted in the school environment?
9. Does the student attend school regularly?
10. Does he/she squint, blink, close or cover one eye at either close or distant viewing tasks?
11. During reading, is there a tendency to skip words, insert incorrect words or guess at words?
12. Does the student use a finger frequently to keep his/her place during reading?
13. Does the student frequently lose his/her place during reading?
14. Is there a tendency to tilt the head during reading?
15. Does the student draw in closer than 10 inches when reading?
16. Is there a tendency for one eye to turn in or out during reading?
17. Is there a considerable head movement during reading?
18. Is there a tendency to vocalize during reading?
19. Does the student develop red eyes or encrusted lids (exclusive of instances of infection)?
20. Does the student complain frequently about reading and study tasks being too time consuming?

Figure 4.17

a vision specialist for a complete visual examination (which hopefully will include evaluations of dynamic functioning).

1. Fixation/Regression Difference Between the Two Eyes–While some differences are undoubtedly attributable to the discernibility of interfixation saccades as influenced by interpupillary dis-

tance alignment of the goggles and the differences that normally exist in the reflectivity of the two eyes, it is estimated that a difference over 1 or 2 percent would probably exceed normal sensor and algorithm variations and should be studied further. Presently, differences over 10 percent in fixations and 20 percent in regressions would seem to warrant further investigation. This condition might especially be significant when the original graphs for both eyes display very similar lengths of return sweeps.

2. Cross Correlation–This data indicates the degree to which the interfixational saccades of the two eyes are similar in excursion throughout the reading. A perfect correlation would be 1.000. Less than this would indicate some degree of difference in the similarity of saccades of the two eyes in either interfixation movement and/or return sweeps. The significance of low correlation is to be studied; probably correlation less than .90 is suspect.
3. Excessive Saccades in Return Sweeps–An excessive number of saccades in return sweep movement could suggest that a subject has incorporated a number of compensating right-to-left movements during or following the execution of a return sweep to achieve proper initial reading location on new lines of print. Inaccuracy in executing return sweeps as evidenced by multiple return sweeps may have been caused by poor vergence/coordination or poor tracking. If return sweeps exceed the lines detected by more than 50 percent, there is cause for concern.
4. Anomalies–This data suggests instances in which the two eyes are not performing in a like manner. Instances in which one eye moved in a forward or reverse manner and the other eye did not move, or instances in which both eyes moved in opposite directions (to be confirmed by examining the Original Graph) are red flags. If any of these numbers exceed four, there may be coordination or vergence difficulties.
5. Original Graph–Beyond the data automatically generated by the Visagraph, further manual inspections of the Original Graph by vision specialists could reveal unusual variations in vergence, loss of binocular control, or any lack of coordination precision in executing return sweeps or interfixation movements. A significant change in the horizontal distance between the plot of the right and left eyes in the Original Graph could indicate a loss of binocular control. A variation in the angularity of fixations at intervals

could indicate a change or accommodation in vergence or fusion. Overshoots or undershoots in the excursions of interfixation saccades or return sweeps would probably signal difficulty in ocular control and/or motility.

In many instances, a school may be reluctant to refer a student to a vision specialist based on Visagraph recording data or his or her comments about visual discomfort. This is unfortunate and not in the best interest of the student who demonstrates excessive difficulty with binocular coordination. The cost of going to a vision specialist to secure visual training should be worked out in the best interest of the student.

CONCLUSION

As you can see from this description of the process of eye movement recording, the performance data derived can be extremely helpful in selecting students for silent reading fluency development practice and planning a program of individualized reading practice. Further, recording eye movements can help evaluate the nature of the changes that have occurred and determine the likelihood that these changes will become permanent or continue to improve. Also, beyond the area of reading improvement there is the detection of visual coordination problems that can possibly serve as a basis for referring a student to a vision specialist for vision training procedures.

QUESTIONS THAT COULD ARISE AFTER READING THIS CHAPTER

1. Since eye movement recording is the only accurate means of examining the nature of a student's Fundamental Reading Process in terms of fixations, regressions, duration of fixation, and span of recognition, which determine the rate of reading as well as the sequence of visual impressions into short-term memory, why shouldn't every student be offered the potential of eye-movement recording testing?

2. Who should administer a Visagraph test and relate findings to the reading remediation course of study?
3. In terms of permanence of gain in both reading rate and comprehension that typically occur after reading development practice, how can one be assured that these gains are permanent and stable without follow-up eye-movement recording testing?
4. What should be done in terms of referral to a vision specialist when students show signs of significant visual/functional problems in their Visagraph recordings and also when they report visual discomfort?

Chapter 5

USES OF EYE MOVEMENT RECORDING AND READING APPRAISALS

As you can see, eye-movement recording can be an invaluable tool in schools and in adult reading improvement programs. They are useful when surveying silent reading efficiency and diagnosing reading performance efficiency characteristics in preparation for a fluency development program to improve reading efficiency.

An eye-movement recording of reading performance efficiency can be an effective diagnostic tool when used in conjunction with any standardized reading test to evaluate both efficiency and effectiveness improvement.

Based on Taylor's grade level norms, judgments can be made about an individual's need for fluency-building techniques to improve his or her reading efficiency. The following briefly suggests some of the symptoms that could indicate a need for a fluency development program.

- Excessive number of fixations (eye stops) and accompanying reduced span of recognition (amount of words or word parts perceived per eye stop)
- Excessive number of regressions
- Unusually prolonged duration of fixation (length of eye pause)
- Poor directional attack
- Inadequate return sweeps
- Habitual rereading
- Inadequate reading rate
- Poor information processing (comprehension)

Depending on the extent of need for a fluency building program, initial judgments can be made about the types of fluency development procedures to be used (i.e., Guided Reading, Tachistoscopic techniques, vocabulary improvement, and comprehension skill development), the extent of fluency training that should be scheduled per week, and the length of a course of instruction.

As a training program progresses, judgments can also be made about the adequacy of attainment using eye-movement recording in combination with the norms for oculomotor characteristics in relation to the reading rate (with good comprehension) attained or desired. In making a judgment about the adequacy of training, a reading diagnostician should check to be sure the oculomotor characteristics (fixations, regressions, etc.) are commensurate with (or better than) the goal rate achieved towards the end of a fluency-building program. For example, using Table 5.1 of reading performance norms in relation to rate-goal performances that are desirable and which can be attained with fluency training, a fourth grade student should be reading at a rate of 230 words per minute (or higher). At this rate, his or her reading performance characteristics should reflect approximately 100 fixations (or fewer), 19 regressions (or fewer), and an average duration of fixation of .26 seconds (or fewer).

Table 5.1

Reading Performance Characteristics														Advanced				
Grade Level	1	2	3	4	5	6	7	8	9	10	11	12	Col.	1	2	3	4	5
[1]Fixations/100 Words	224	174	155	139	129	120	114	109	105	101	96	94	90	77	65	57	48	44
[2]Regressions/100 Words	52	40	35	31	28	25	23	21	20	19	18	17	15	11	8	5	4	2
Directional Attack %	23	23	23	24	22	21	20	19	19	19	19	18	17	14	12	9	8	5
Av. Span of Recognition	.45	.57	.65	.72	.78	.83	.88	.92	.95	.99	1.04	1.06	1.11	1.30	1.53	1.75	2.08	2.27
Av. Duration of Fixation	.33	.30	.28	.27	.27	.27	.27	.27	.27	.26	.26	.25	.24	.23	.23	.22	.22	.22
Rate without Rereading	80	115	138	158	173	185	195	204	214	224	237	250	280	340	400	480	560	620

Grade Level	1	2	3	4	5	6	7	8	9	10	11	12	Col.
Desirable Goal Rates by Grade or Goal **	140	170	200	230	250	270	280	300	310	325	345	360	400
See above chart for appropriate performance characteristics which are in accord with goal reading rates.													

Likewise an adult whose job responsibilities require a goal reading level competency of grade 12 should be reading at a rate of 360 words per minute (or higher), averaging 77 fixations (or fewer) and 11 regressions (or fewer), and employing an average duration of fixation of .23 seconds (or fewer).

Reading Fluency/Changes in Eye-Movement Performance

The goal of any reading improvement program is not to specifically change eye-movement behavior, but rather to develop adequate levels of efficiency in the Fundamental Reading Process skills, resulting in increased fluency in silent reading in order that students find reading a more successful and enjoyable process. Fluency is defined as reading with ease and comfort at an adequate rate and with good comprehension. If adequate levels of reading fluency are developed, then the eye-movement performance of an individual will, naturally and normally, improve in all characteristics (number of fixations, regressions, span of recognition, etc.). Likewise, there will be an accompanying improvement in the results of any standardized tests administered as a student or trainee becomes a more efficient and effective reader.

At all levels of reading instruction, whether developmental or remedial in nature, Guided Reading (and Tachistoscopic) training techniques should be employed to develop adequate levels of reading fluency in both struggling and achieving student readers. These training methods remain the most expeditious means of developing higher levels of efficiency and fluency in silent reading:

- Flash (tachistoscopic) training with numbers, letters, and words, as shown in Figure 5.1, can improve a student's realization of the orthography of words and the development of greater word recognition automaticity. During these high-speed exposures, only one fixation is possible when the exposures are one-sixth of a second or faster. Increasing the accuracy with which a student identifies letter configurations and developing more instant recognition of words within a single fixation will result in more time and mental capacity for word association, phrasing, and understanding during each duration of fixation.

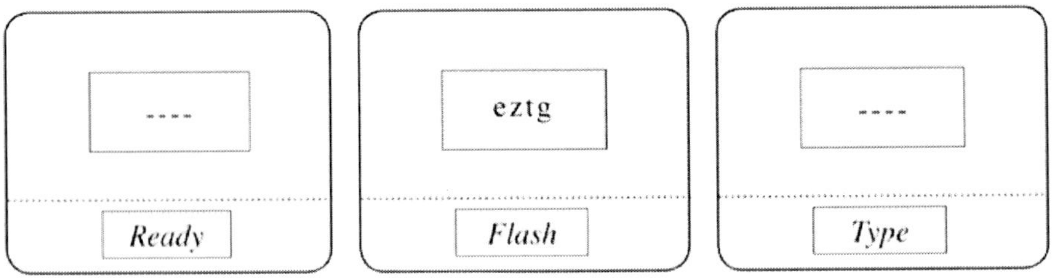

Figure 5.1

- The Guided Reading program, through timed left-to-right displays of print in the manner shown Figure 5.2, where a moving window displays print, can result in a number of changes that will produce improved reading efficiency in both oculomotor behaviors and cognitive function.

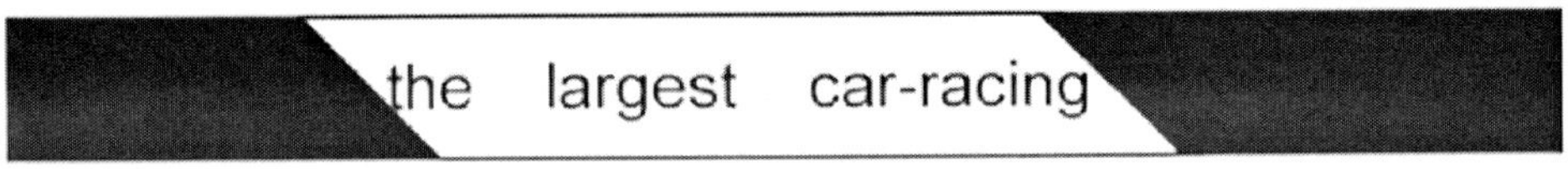

Figure 5.2

The scanning training provided by these left-to-right timed displays of text will have a number of beneficial results. As students read and model their reading behavior in accord with such text displays, the following changes occur:

- Improved visual functioning (binocular coordination), ocular motility (the ability to move the eyes instead of the head), and accuracy in tracking (both horizontally and vertically).
- The faster-than-usual occluding of print from left to right discourages habitual regressions and also eliminates recovery eye movements that typically follow regressions, resulting in improved sequence of word input into short-term memory. Overall, fixations are reduced as the student learns to perceive more rapidly and sequentially.
- Duration of fixation shortens as a result of the brief, timed displays of all words. Word recognition time decreases and greater automaticity is encouraged if the reading content also provides fre-

quent repetition of high-frequency vocabulary through shorter, timed displays of each word.
- Students are encouraged to direct more of their attention to the right of their fixation point, which increases the potential for them to use parafoveal letter and word clues to better guide upcoming saccadic excursions.
- The unveiling of words in a left-to-right fashion enhances the potential for improved orthographic awareness, and the timed closing down of word displays discourages slower conscious attention to decoding and encourages more rapid word recognition.
- Some risk-taking in word perception is encouraged, which allows the student to proceed with continuous reading, and later to confirm recognition of encountered words during phrasing and to confirm meaning through the use of the context that follows.
- Comprehension improves as students input words more rapidly and sequentially into short-term memory as comprehension questions guide the students to more global and thorough comprehension.

Reading development systems, such as Reading Plus, flash, Guided Reading, and SeeReader program techniques (in which timed left-to-right displays of text are employed) form the foundation for developing the visual/functional, perceptual, and information-processing skills that determine a student's reading fluency and his or her oculomotor efficiency.

Primary Grades/Beginning Reading Adults

In the primary grades or in a program of adult literacy for beginning readers, a reading fluency development program should be part of an ongoing beginning reading curriculum on a weekly basis to ensure the following:

- High levels of attention and concentration
- Efficient visual/functional skills
- Good directional attack
- Heightened visual discrimination
- Strong visual memory

- Instantaneous word recognition
- Rapid word association
- Improved phrasing
- Heightened comprehension
- Adequate reading rate

This author (1981) conducted research from 1978 to1981 with 1,335 first and second grade students in 56 schools to demonstrate that instrument-based fluency building techniques, used as recommended with basal reading instruction, allowed students to attain reading rates with good comprehension that were commensurate or higher than their usual oral speech range (125 to 175 wpm). The reading rates achieved by trained students were significantly (<.01) greater than those evidenced by non-trained students. The reading rates of the students in this study are shown in the Table 5.2.

Table 5.2

Taylor Grade 1 - 2 Study Group			
Grade	Mean Normative Rate (Standard eye movement reading tests)	Mean Pre-Testing Rates (Basal reading content)	Mean Post-Testing Rates (Basal and standardized training content)
1	80 wpm	104 wpm	143-158 wpm
2	115 wpm	140 wpm	164-179 wpm
3	138	143-164	

A 2006 study of second grade students by Shelley-Tremblay and Eyer (2009) showed the impact that fluency in silent reading development techniques can have on oculomotor and perceptual development. The second grade students engaged in Reading Plus programs for a semester, involving both flash and Guided Reading training. Table 5.3 displays the contrast between the normative performance of second graders (Taylor et al., 1960) and the performance of second graders who received a semester of fluency development training. This eye-movement data was secured at mid-year for both the normative performance and the fluency training group.

Further, the Gates-MacGinitie NCE growth in test scores for the treatment group was 1.4 years in contrast to the gain of the non-training group, which was only .7 years.

Table 5.3

Grade 2 Taylor Normative Performance / Fluency Training Performance		
	Normative Performance	Following Fluency Training
Fixations	174	152 (155 is norm for 3rd graders)
Regressions	57	26 (25 is norm for 6th graders)
Reading Rates	115 wpm	150 wpm (158 is norm for 4th graders

Intermediate Grades and Higher

During the intermediate grade levels and higher, the development of silent reading fluency should be one of the initial concerns in any reading improvement program, whether remedial, corrective, or developmental. Regardless of the reading achievement level of a student or trainee, his or her fluency level, in terms of Fundamental Reading Process competencies, should be raised to the rate and performance shown in Table 5.4.

In general, it is expected that a student engaged in fluency development practice will achieve more efficient reading, reflected in a higher rate of reading.

Table 5.4

Grade Level	1	2	3	4	5	6	7	8	9	10	11	12	Col.
1960 Norm Reading Rates by Grade	80	115	138	158	17	185	195	204	214	224	237	250	280
Desirable Goal Rates by Grade or Goal	140	170	200	230	250	270	280	300	310	325	345	360	400

During the process of fluency training, a student or trainee will evidence improvement in the following:

- Ability to focus and sustain attention
- Increased ease and comfort during reading
- Improved oculomotor efficiency in reading
- Improved vocabulary
- More rapid, accurate, and orderly reading of content

- Increased ability to read and remember more from a single visual encounter
- Ability to associate ideas more rapidly and effectively

In a study by Schlange, Patel, and Caden (1999), sixth and eighth grade students, judged to be at risk in terms of academic failure, were enrolled in a Reading Plus program for only a two-month period. Students using Reading Plus statistically exceeded the gain over "paired" non-participants on the Iowa Tests of Basic Skills scores. Additionally, Visagraph eye-movement recording pre- and post-examinations revealed significant improvement in oculomotor performance in terms of a reduction in students' number of fixations, regressions, and durations of fixation, while at the same time improving their reading rates significantly. Beyond this, students who participated in Reading Plus demonstrated considerable improvement in binocular coordination as measured in 12 different visual performance areas.

Once a student or trainee has achieved a reasonable and satisfactory level of reading fluency, he or she is better prepared to acquire more complex strategies of contextual analysis, more advanced comprehension skills, job or content area reading strategies, skimming and scanning approaches, etc. In fact all of these more complex reading skills presume, and indeed require, an adequate level of basic silent reading fluency to emerge successfully.

As a student or trainee, at any level, becomes a more fluent reader, significant changes occur in oculomotor and perceptual behavior, which reflect in his or her physical ease and comfort, as well as rate and comprehension during reading. When eye-movement recordings are taken before, during, and following such fluency development training activities, there will always be a significant change in the following oculomotor or eye-movement performance:

- Reduction of fixations
- Reduction of regressions
- Increase in average span of recognition
- Decrease in average duration of fixation (if unnecessarily prolonged initially)
- Increase in reading rate with good comprehension
- Improvement in visual/functional competence

CONCLUSION

There is no doubt that the Fundamental Reading Process skills involving a reader's visual/functional competence, perceptual accuracy and efficiency, and information-processing capability are the most basic of reading skills that determine the degree with which silent reading is a fluent and efficient process. It is essential that a student's level of competency in these skills be assessed, and to date, the only means of evaluating the level of these skills is through eye-movement recording. With today's dedication to have all students demonstrate competence in all areas of learning through a common core curriculum, it seems logical that all students should be tested with eye-movement recording to ensure that their basic visual, perceptual, and information-processing skills are sufficiently efficient to allow silent reading to become a comfortable, satisfying, and rewarding activity. This accomplishment is essential if reading is to serve the need for advanced studies and to achieve vocational competency.

With today's stress on achieving common core standards, which largely focus on advanced vocabulary and comprehension skills, it is critical not to lose sight of the basic need to develop meaningful competency in the fundamental reading-process skills that initiate all forms of reading. Without meaningful competency in the visual/functional, perceptual, and information-processing skills, more advanced readers will still experience considerable difficulty in achieving meaningful reading rates and the ease of reading that is required for advanced studies. In many cases, a lack of fundamental skills will result in less comfortable reading, slower reading rates, and the need to reread excessively.

Eye movement recording can provide the following critical information regarding silent reading:

- Reflections of reading efficiency
- Predictions about reading effectiveness
- Reflections of visual/functional, perceptual, and cognitive adaptations over time

QUESTIONS THAT COULD ARISE AFTER READING THIS CHAPTER

1. Since the nature of the basic visual and perceptual performance skills are widely documented today in research literature, why would eye-movement recording not be used to accurately measure the oculomotor efficiency of all students, especially struggling readers or students who are reading at very slow rates?
2. What other reading development activities should be implemented, along with such activities as flash training and guided reading practice, to achieve even more comprehensive gains in silent reading fluency development?

Chapter 6

VISAGRAPH FIELD USE–SCHOOLS

This chapter will explain the various settings in which the Visagraph eye-movement recording system has been used in schools, clinics, and by vision specialists. Additionally, users will be provided with guidelines in terms of the effective use of eye-movement recording techniques.

The use of eye-movement recording with the Visagraph will naturally vary in terms of students to be tested, the frequency of testing, and the level of the test selections to be employed based on the testing situation. Schools may use the Visagraph selectively with various types of students, whereas reading clinics will typically use the Visagraph with most all students and will principally vary the testing and re-testing routine in relation to their instructional schedules. Likewise, optometrists who are providing visual/functional training to improve reading, as well as general visual competence, will use the Visagraph testing with most clients, but perhaps in a slightly different manner and at more frequent intervals during their visual training procedures.

ELEMENTARY, MIDDLE, AND SECONDARY SCHOOL ASSESSMENTS

Schools may choose to use the Visagraph to select which students need to be enrolled in a fluency-training program such as Reading Plus, or they may decide to test entire grades to make sure the students are adequately prepared for the reading challenges ahead of them. As an example, a large metropolitan city may be utilizing a large number of Visagraphs with many of their schools. During an initial orientation, teachers who will manage the Visagraph testing in each school should be trained as Visagraph testing specialists and then these teachers will decide in concert with the administration which students are to be tested and how frequently. For example, one goal might be to test all fourth graders to be sure that those in need of fluency development receive early training, so that their reading competency is assured in preparation for the intermediate grades' science, social studies, math, reading, and study needs.

Or an evaluation may be made on the basis of standardized test scores in order that those students who exhibit the greatest need for silent reading fluency development are accommodated first and in the most intensive manner. Or the decision may be that all ninth grade students might be assessed in preparation for selecting students who exhibit the greatest need for fluency development in their secondary studies.

Or the decision may be made to focus on those students classified as exhibiting special needs and to schedule more intensive use of Reading Plus five times a week to make sure that they are returned to adequate silent reading fluency performances.

Or students may be selected on the basis of their feelings about their reading competency. It is imperative that students who feel that reading is an unsuccessful chore be focused on as soon as possible. Their outlook in terms of their reading in the various subject areas will be more successful and they will believe they can make major improvements using Reading Plus.

Next is the frequency of testing or retesting to be decided upon in conjunction with the Reading Plus System. Testing may occur at the beginning and end of a trimester or semester. Some students may be retested after every 10 to 20 sessions to ensure their progress is encouraging, and if not as expected, to increase the frequency of training or to make other program adjustments to ensure adequate gains.

For larger school implementations, as mentioned above, it is recommended to assign lead Visagraph specialists (e.g., teachers) who will coordinate the Visagraph testing, interpret the testing results, and help make decisions regarding all Reading Plus scheduling.

Guidelines for Visagraph Testing

- Time–When planning for Visagraph testing, allow seven to 10 minutes per student so there is time for a retest if comprehension is not satisfactory or if a low cross correlation suggests the need for a confirming retest. It is likely that only six students per hour can be tested. Based on this basic scheduling, the number of students should be planned for per day. This testing might extend into the period of time in which students are engaged in the early stages of Reading Plus usage.

- Testing Location–It is advisable to test in one room with students waiting in an adjacent room so as to expedite the Visagraph testing. As one student completes testing, the next student should immediately report for testing. Students who are waiting for their turn for their Visagraph test should bring some reading or study material to occupy their wait time.
- Advanced Determination of the Level of Visagraph Test to Be Used–It will expedite testing if students have taken the Reading Plus Reading Placement Appraisal™ which will auto-assign students to the proper Visagraph test level. If other tests are going to be used to determine the appropriate test level, this should be done well in advance of the actual Visagraph testing to expedite matters.

Frequency of Use of the Visagraph

Visagraph testing can be used at various intervals for various purposes:

1. Retesting might occur after students complete 5, 10, 15, 30, 45, or 60 Reading Plus lessons to be sure that adequate and steady progress in silent reading fluency is being achieved.
2. Retesting might be scheduled to revise the nature of Reading Plus weekly training schedules.
3. Retesting might be used to determine whether some different forms of fluency-development training might be warranted. For example, the use of pre-reading approaches could be scheduled if students are encountering difficulty in maintaining good comprehension when rate is increased or when higher level content is encountered.
4. Post-testing should always be scheduled to determine the probability of fluency gains being maintained.

5. Retesting might be scheduled if there is a concern that a student might need to be referred to a vision specialist for VT training.

College Level Use

Silent reading fluency development and the Visagraph are also used in many college-level programs. Obviously, a college student is more advanced academically but might still lack meaningful proficiency in the basic visual/functional, perceptual, and informational processing skills to be a truly efficient reader. As a result, many college students are slow and labored in their rate of reading and somewhat limited in terms of comprehension. The report that follows is typical of the Visagraph use in a college-level program.

Northeastern Junior College, Sterling, Colorado

The lead teacher who supervised the Visagraph testing and the use of Reading Plus is Maret Felzien, MA, Reading Specialist/Associate Professor at Northeastern Junior College, a two-year public, comprehensive community college serving approximately 1,500 full-time and 4,000 part-time students. The population is drawn from many remote and small high schools but also attracts students from cities and out of state.

In over a decade of use, the college has employed Visagraph testing and Reading Plus programs in their remedial courses and provided results-based information on a number of occasions through the years. Additionally, parents bring their school-aged children to the college for Visagraph testing as a way of gaining additional information when they are struggling with *why* a child isn't thriving at school. Also the local eye-doctor/vision therapist uses the college as a resource, specifically requesting pre/post Visagraph screenings to give them information they cannot otherwise gather.

A Visagraph assessment is scheduled approximately twice during the school year and they follow the general guidelines described here.

Currently, Northeastern offers three levels of remedial reading. The Visagraph is consistently used in the highest-level remedial reading course, and periodically (due to time limitations) in their two lower-level courses. At the highest level, the Visagraph is used at the beginning of the one-semester course where students work on Guided

Reading during the semester with a goal of reaching 40 or more stories in their training. At the end of the semester, 15 to 16 weeks later, students are reassessed using the Visagraph.

The Visagraph is used here in two ways: as a secondary/tertiary assessment for placement into courses and as an effective motivator for students.

ASSESSMENT–When students, who are initially tested with Accuplacer, test at a higher level on the Visagraph and individual questioning and tutoring indicate that they can work beyond the level of their Accuplacer placement, the Visagraph data is used as support to validate changing placement.

MOTIVATION–Northeastern's Reading Specialist, Maret Felzien, reports that motivation is a primary reason for her use of the Visagraph, particularly with the highest-level group:

> I focus on the highest-level reading course because I see the most students in these classes, and they spend the most time with me (16 vs. 8 weeks). My theory is that I can teach good reading practices until I am blue in the face, but until we really begin to address their basic reading skills, only so much gain can be made. By sharing the results of the Visagraph with each of the students and explaining what it means about their reading (and showing how their reading can change over time), they begin to understand what they can work on to improve their skills AND it helps to explain *why* they have struggled with reading for so long. This helps with buy-in, motivation, and also self-awareness. By following up with a post Visagraph, students get to see first hand the specific changes they have experienced. This is a really powerful moment. Not only do they realize that their reading has vastly improved (and they will talk about how reading is easier, or quicker, or they find they understand more, etc.), but then they can see it demonstrated for them on their pre/post Visagraph tests. The look of accomplishment on their faces, not to mention the sense of validation, is worth the effort.

A study at Northeastern Junior College in 2000 involved students in two remedial courses in which they were placed using Accuplacer. Students in the lower course (REA 060) scored reading levels in the grades four through eight ranges, while students in the higher course (REA 90) scored in the grades nine through 11 ranges.

Pre- and post-tests were done using the Visagraph II Eye Movement Recording System. Visagraph post-tests were used to assess changes in the efficiency of the Fundamental Reading Process for each student.

Students received classroom instruction two days per week and also engaged in Guided Reading and PAVE™ once a week in the laboratory for eight weeks. Each student worked to complete an average of 40 Guided Reading stories. PAVE was used for about eight minutes per session.

Average pre-test/post-test recording data provides measured components of the Fundamental Reading Process. This data reflects the following information:

- Fixations (number of eye stops per 100 words)
- Regressions (number of reverse eye movements per 100 words)
- Average Duration of Fixation (in milliseconds)
- Rate of Reading with Comprehension (in words per minute)
- Grade Level Equivalent (according to national norms)
- Directional Attack Difficulty (difficulty with characteristic tendency to perceive and organize content in a left-to-right manner)

Pre- and post-test averages from the Visagraph Profile data for 30 college-level students in REA 060 remedial class (grouped data for three classes) during the year 2000 are displayed in Table 6.1. Similar results continue to be achieved.

Table 6.1

30 College-Level Students REA 060 Remedial						
Grade	Fixations	Regressions	Duration of Fixation	Rate of Reading (wpm) with Comprehension	Grade Level Equivalent	Directional Attack Difficulty
Pre-Test	122	15	270	191	7.0	12
Post-Test	98	10	267	245	10.2	10
Change	Improved by 24 or 20%	Improved by 5 or 33%	Improved by 3 ms	Improved by 54 or 22%	Improved by 3.5 or 33%	Improved by 2

Pre- and post-test averages from the Visagraph Profile data for 44 college-level students in REA 090 remedial class are displayed in Talbe 6.2.

Results yielded substantial increases of 3.5 (33 percent) and 4.2 (34 percent) in respective classes in Grade Level Efficiency, as measured by the Visagraph, along with improvements in all components of the Fundamental Reading Process in all classes. Although the higher-level

Table 6.2

44 College-Level Students REA 090 Remedial						
Grade	Fixations	Regressions	Duration of Fixation	Rate of Reading (wpm) with Comprehension	Grade Level Equivalent	Directional Attack Difficulty
Pre-Test	119	17	250	191	8.3	14
Post-Test	86	8	244	245	12.5	9
Change	Improved by 33 or 28%	Improved by 9 or 33%	Improved by 6 ms	Improved by 99 or 32%	Improved by 4.2 or 34%	Improved by 5

remedial group exhibited slightly greater improvement in most characteristics, both groups demonstrated significant changes overall. Fixations in both groups decreased by an impressive one-third.

The overall improvements in all measures of oculomotor performance suggested that instruction with Reading Plus is an effective means of improving reading efficiency for college-level students. In addition the reading specialist indicated that the program was a positive experience for the students and that Reading Plus and the Visagraph were important components of the remedial program. Because the results of this study are so positive, Reading Plus and the Visagraph should become a regular part of college-level reading development programs.

In a more recent study, Northeastern Junior College was one of nine schools participating in the longitudinal component of a national research project conducted by Dr. John Shelley-Tremblay of the University of South Alabama, Department of Psychology. This portion of the study involved college students enrolled in remedial reading courses. The students involved made substantial gains on their Accu- placer scores, improving by an average of 26 percent over their preliminary assessment scores. This included 57 students who engaged in Reading Plus activities for one semester and five who continued for two semesters. The students who continued on showed much greater gains on average than did those who were in the program for a semester. A remarkable one semester gain was also seen in the 25 students who were both pre- and post-tested using the Visagraph Eye Movement Recording System. They improved their reading efficiency by an average of 4.6 Grade Level Equivalents in a single semester. The expected improvement over a year without specific training is 1.0 GLEs. Within the Reading Plus system, the students improved their Part B, or guided slot, rate by an average of 92 percent while maintaining an average comprehension of 70 percent or more over an average of 43 lessons.

Poplar Bluff Kindergarten Center Vision Intervention Program Data, 2007–2008

The Visagaraph has also been used with kindergarten students not yet involved in reading as a means to explore whether their visual/functional skills will permit satisfactory reading instruction. Following is one study conducted in Kansas with kindergarten students to make sure that the students involved in the study were prepared for reading instruction.

Purpose of Review

This review was conducted to discover if a correlation existed between the Learning Insights manual visual/functional screening assessment and the Taylor Associates' Visagraph III Eye Movement Assessment, in a kindergarten population. The team wanted specifically to examine the correlation between the two assessments in the area of binocular coordination: vergence, ocular motility, and accuracy in tracking.

Background

Well-developed visual/functional abilities prepare beginning students for success in their school experience. Learning to read and reading for information require efficient visual abilities; the eyes must team precisely, focus clearly, and track quickly and accurately across a page of print. By the end of third grade, students are expected to read independently and proficiently. By providing early identification and intervention, appropriate perceptual skill development will occur.

Just as public schools conduct vision and hearing screenings, Learning Insights' Vision Intervention Program (VIP) screens kindergarten through third grade students' visual/ functional skills. Through the VIP assessment, almost 15,000 kindergarten through third graders have been screened. Results have demonstrated that 41 percent of these children have visional/ functional issues. The VIP trains and certifies school personnel to manually screen students and then they provide tutoring to students who demonstrated visional/functional delays.

The Visagrap III (VG-III), developed by Taylor Associates, has gained recognition by the College of Optometrists in Vision Development (COVD) and is used in many optometry offices across the nation to assess visual/ functional impairments. The VG-III technology is also utilized in thousands of schools. The VG-III is used most commonly with students in first grade through adulthood. It provides information in the areas of reading, functional vision, visual simulations of eye-movements, and graphs that depict specific details of visual coordination. The VG-III is part of the Reading Plus silent fluency reading program which has changed reading habits and enhanced visual perception in struggling readers.

Perceptual issues require immediate identification and remediation in order for a student to become a proficient learner. When remediation is not provided, students become struggling readers and develop other academic deficits. Often students with visual/functional delays display behaviors that falsely label them as ADHD, dyslexic, behavior problems, and apathetic. These students are often placed in remedial or special education programs where they spend years making slow and arduous progress, losing self-esteem and confidence each day. Unresolved visual deficits are certain to impair the ability to respond fully to educational instruction and require early intervention.

Population

The Poplar Bluff Kindergarten Center (PBKC) in Poplar Bluff, Missouri, was chosen for the correlation review because of its diverse population. The PBKC housed approximately 400 kindergarten students that represented rural and city dwellers, five ethnic groups, and all income levels. The students were first screened manually with the VIP five-point assessment. From that screening 128 students were identified as having one or all of the following visual/functional issues: Visual Pursuit (tracking), Cover Test/Alternate Cover-Uncover Test (eye-teaming), Saccades (motility), Near Point Convergence (vergence), and Form Reproduction. Then all VIP students were screened using the Visagraph III eye-movement assessment. Finally the data was reviewed to determine if a positive correlation existed between the two screening instruments.

Implementation

The 128 VIP students were individually assessed with the Visagraph III. The room was prepared by posting photos of children wearing the VG-III goggles; kindergarten-sized seating was provided and arranged to avoid window glare or white backgrounds.

The following procedure ensued:

Students were brought into the room in pairs; this eased the anxiety of the students in this new situation and allowed the examiner to explain the procedure to both students at once. The students were shown the goggles which were explained to them in children's' terms. Then the students were shown the VG-III booklet, specifically the Visual Skills and the Numbers pages, and the directions were reviewed. After instruction, one student sat at a table with an activity while the other student completed the assessment.

- Step 1–The goggles were secured to the student's head with a Velcro strap; in most cases this was adequate. Children who had small heads were fitted with the goggles, then three-inch strips of gray foam were placed at the edge of the goggles where it aligned with the temple. This was done to provide comfort and to prevent too much light from entering the recording. The goggles were slightly oversized for some students; however, all students were able to utilize them with the above adjustments. The students were provided with a mirror in order to view themselves with the goggles. Every attempt was made to ensure the students felt comfortable interacting with the assessment tools. Final adjustments were made to the IPD settings.
- Step 2–Student were presented with the VG-III booklet again. The Visual Skills Test, designed to record and analyze a student's performance in fixation maintenance (convergence) and motility (saccades) were presented in age-appropriate language. Students were directed to only use their eyes because this was an eye game.

When students moved their heads, lips, or mouths, they were reminded that only the eyes were to play this game so please keep the rest of the body still. Many students had difficulty with this, but after a few tries most of the recordings were deemed acceptable for data review. In the Visual Skills assessment, the examiner often pointed to the X displayed in the booklet, or moved her finger between the Xs to demonstrate the desired movement.

- Step 3–The student was then presented the Numbers Test. This test is also used with non-readers or beginning readers. They do not have to say the numbers, they only have to look at each number, and thus tracking may be observed, as well as binocular coordination and vergence. Many students had difficulty with this task. The student was allowed to try this task without assistance but more often than not, the examiner used her finger to move from number to number. The majority of the students were able to complete these assessments with the described support.

Overt student behaviors were noted on the protocol. Observations included movement of mouth or jaw as students completed the Visual Skills motility Test. When completing the Numbers Test, there was movement of lips or mouth and at times eyes watered or became itchy.

Summary of Findings

The Visagraph III was not specifically designed for use with kindergarten students; however, it has shown itself to be an adaptable and dependable, easy-to-use tool. This review clearly indicated a positive correlation between the VG-III and the VIP manual screening processes. Utilizing the scores from the VG-III kindergarten Screening form in comparison to the manual VIP assessment results, a positive correlation was established. The VG-III, Visual Skills Test, analyzed performance in fixation maintenance (vergence) and motility (saccades). When this data was compared to the VIP data of convergence and saccades, a positive correlation was evidenced. Approximately 85 percent of the kindergarten students displayed significantly low visual/functional scores on both instruments. This indicated the students were having a difficult time focusing (vergence) on a fixed target for 15 seconds and were unable to rhythmically complete saccades (motility) for 20 seconds. The VG-III Numbers data was then compared to the VIP Tracking data, which indicated approximately 75 percent correlation. The examiner believed this correlation was slightly lower because assistance was provided as the examiner pointed to the target when the student was unable to complete the task independently.

Ninety-three of the 128 students identified with visual/functional issues completed the VIP intervention tutoring. Tutoring consisted of 20-minute sessions twice a week that provided convergence, tracking, and motility activities. Ninety-seven percent of the VIP students obtained kindergarten DIBELS scores at, or above, the scores of students who received no vision intervention tutoring.

This review demonstrated that the VG-III can be utilized to gain valuable information concerning kindergarten students visual/functional needs and correlated positively with an established manual screening. The VG-III was also able to provide printable information and graphs depicting eye-movement, which were utilized by parents and optometrists. Additional information can be obtained by contacting the following:

- Vision Intervention Program, Learning Insights, 11560 Fletcher Lane, Holts Summit, MO 65043, www.goodvision4all.org. Contact: Michael Flynn, Director, 573–291–1187
- Poplar Bluff R-1 Kindergarter Center, 1235 N. Main, Poplar Bluff, MO, 63901, phaeton@pb.k12.mo.us. Contact: Pam Heaton, Director of VIP at Kindergarten Center, 573–785–7751
- Taylor Associates Communications, Inc. 110 West Canal Street, Suite 301, Winooski, VT, 05404, www.readingplus.com. Contact: Alexandra Spichtig, Director of Product Development, 802–735–1942/800–549–3000
- School District Improvement Programs, LLC, 616 Pine Cone Rd, Poplar Bluff, MO, 63901, kennedy.sheri@gmail.com. Contact: Sheri Kennedy, School Psychological Examiner, 573–686–4240

Douglas County, Colorado

The section that follows is a discussion on January 30, 2012 with Holly Voorhees Carmical who is the Curriculum Coordinator for Douglas County, Colorado. In her role as Curriculum Coordinator for the District, she focuses on literacy and social studies. She works in both elementary and secondary schools.

Holly holds a Master's Degree (M.A.) in Education. She is currently working toward completing her doctorate in Educational Leadership.

Although most schools that have the Visagraph have constant access to it, the section that follows indicates how in Douglas County, Colorado they share only four Visagraph units with loans to approximately 30 to 45 schools within the county.

Conversation with Holly Voorhees Carmical

How frequently is a Visagraph loaned to an individual school and for how long a time period?

Schools request Visagraph units all the time. The four machines are checked out constantly to a variety of schools–elementary, middle, and high. When schools borrow it, they keep it for a week to Visagraph most of their Reading Plus students. They focus predominantly on the students who were a puzzle to them. Over 50 schools have access to the Visagraph; between 30 and 35 schools in the district have utilized the Visagraph at some point.

At times, specific schools request to have me come out to Visagraph students for them. For example, one of the Reading Recovery teachers in the district has me Visagraph her puzzle students–the students who are still a mystery to her as a trained Reading Recovery teacher. At times, I have administered a Visa- graph test on nonreaders who were not yet old enough for Reading Plus.

Do they have a goal in mind for their use of the Visagraph?

Yes. Approximately two to three years ago, I started working with Occupational Therapists. The Visagraph is used in conjunction with an IEP as a piece of information that can assist in providing a whole picture of the student as a learner. Teachers who are trained in using the Visagraph check it out quite a bit. Smaller schools will call me to come out and administer the Visagraph tests. Many of the schools want to Visagraph students who are not necessarily on Reading

Plus, especially at the elementary school level. It's the kids who are presenting issues and teachers and other professionals want to understand what could be going on. They are generally focusing on administering a Visagraph test on the kids who are struggling with reading.

One school started using Reading Plus after they had experience with the Visagraph. The Visagraph is also used as a tool to help students understand how they take in text and how this impacts comprehension. I suspect that schools use the Visagraph as a teaching tool for teachers as well-it is something that shows teachers how students take in text. The Visagraph has actually changed the way teachers view certain students. The students are no longer seen as lazy-teachers understand more of the student's experience. This is an eye-opening experience for the teachers.

Who would be the person who is going to administer the Visagraph testing in each school?

I try to train just one person at a school. This is typically the Building Resource Teacher or the Reading Plus Lead Teacher. Sometimes, I train the SPED teacher. It is different at various schools. The trained teacher often trains other people at the school and it gets spread around. I try to keep it at a limited number of people because sometimes I get Visagraph units returned broken or with parts missing because it wasn't packaged correctly. Teachers do get excited and want to share. Typically, the person who gets trained is the one who originally brought Reading Plus to the school (the Building Resource Teacher or the Reading Plus Lead Teacher).

What would be the goal of the responsible person?

The goal is to get information for the teachers who are requesting it and to inform teachers about how students are taking in text. Part of the other goal might be to answer the following questions: should this child be on Reading Plus; are there other modifications we need to make for the student?

When one particular school first started using Visagraph, the teachers there were able to identify a kindergartner with extreme eye tracking issues. The school contacted a vision therapist and got a home therapy package ($300) to use with the child at school. They went through the home vision therapy program with this young student to change the way she tracked. Now she is in second grade and doing well. If they had not been able to catch the issue with the Visagraph, she would have been a student who would have struggled for years. It was such a benefit to figure it out at such a young age.

Schools within the district have screened a lot of kindergartners in order to catch things early with respect to tracking.

How is the Visagraph data related to the use of the Reading Plus system?

Typically, schools will Visagraph students who are already using Reading Plus to see how they are taking in text. The data gives the teacher more information and brings a huge level of awareness to teachers using the program. Sometimes the information is used to put kids on Reading Plus. Teachers have used PAVE with levels K, 1, and 2; they have also used Word Memory and DeCode with first grader students. They try to start building capacity with non-readers who are not yet ready for Reading Plus.

Older students are shown their Visagraph recordings to demystify their challenges. Many times, I have heard, "You need to show that to my mom. I'm not dumb." Recordings are used to show kids and teachers data. They are also using data to place students into Reading Plus. Placement into the program is not random. When teachers ask, "What do we do with the student?" We say, "Put them on Reading Plus." There are vision therapists in the county who use Reading Plus as a part of their intervention within the clinic setting. It is a huge benefit that Douglas County is offering this to students at their schools. I am not a program person, but this is an amazing program.

One story from Sagewood Middle School: Every single sixth grader was on the program last year and their reading scores this year are incredible. If everyone is in the program, the program will do its job.

How many schools in Douglas County are using the Visagraph?

Approximately 30 to 35 schools have used the Visagraph over the past few years. There are perhaps some schools that have purchased their own Visagraph, but I don't know for certain how many. I often hear teachers say, "We want one of our own." There are "frequent flyer" schools that use it all the time.

Is the Visagraph used by elementary schools more frequently than intermediate and secondary schools? Is it used with particular populations more than others (struggling readers only, specific grade levels, for example)?

It is used by more elementary than secondary schools. We have more elementary schools, but it's still proportionately higher. Elementary schools want it all the time to help understand their reading problem issues. By middle school, students have an ILP and the issues have been identified already in elementary. Predomin- antly, the Visagraph is used in first and second grade. Students are hitting a challenge and teachers want to understand why. When I'm called in, it's for K and first grade, perhaps secondary level by virtue of time-period-based requests in the beginning of the school year.

If a student is administered a Visagraph test, is he or she retested again after a certain interval of time?

This is typically the case at the secondary level. Teachers of older students love the pre- and post-assessment picture. Time interval seems pretty random in the elementary schools as they Visagraph at odd times. Middle school and high school is beginning of year and end of year. The pre- and post- is more prevalent in middle and high schools.

Please share any anecdotes or other pieces of information regarding the use of the Visagraph within Douglas County. Is there anything else you would like to see in print?

I love the story of the kindergartner who had a major issue that was caught very early. I also like the fact that in Douglas County, there is a team of OTs working closely with the Visagraph data to combine solutions with Reading Plus. OTs are able to provide additional activities that build tracking (activities outside of Reading

Plus).

Who would have thought we could find out this information about kids and to use it to really make a difference in their lives? The Visagraph shows so much more than you could ever really see. It shifts people's minds and shifts the way people think about their students.

QUESTIONS THAT COULD ARISE AFTER READING THIS CHAPTER

1. How might a comprehensive Visagraph testing program be successfully employed in a traditional school setting?
2. Who should be in charge of such testing programs?
3. How frequently should students be retested with the Visagraph?
4. How would the Visagraph results help determine reading remediation programs, especially in silent reading development programs?

Chapter 7

VISAGRAPH FIELD USE–READING CLINICS

Many reading clinics throughout the United States use the Visagraph to ensure a more thorough reading appraisal, as well as a more accurate evaluation resulting from their reading remediation. Following are some reports from clinics.

Stacy Dean, President
Dean's Learning Center
Hamilton, New Jersey
Phone: 609–585–1274
Cell: 609–439–1669
stacy@deanslearningcenter.com

I'd like to provide you with a little background information on Dean's Learning Center (DLC). The majority of our students are from low-income families and receive our tutoring program through their Title I school district as part of Supplemental Educational Services (SES). Our students vary in age (grades K–12), race, and ability, and many receive special education, basic skills, or ESL services within their school. I'm sharing this information with you because I think it will make our results even more amazing!

We try to give a Visagraph test to every student who will use Reading Plus. However, there are some circumstances where we just don't have the time to complete Visagraph testing on everyone. Therefore we focus on the older students within the group first.

We test the students at their initial assessment level based upon their results of the Reading Placement Appraisal (Form A). Then students are given a second Visagraph test at their post-assessment level, once they have completed the program. Completion means they have used all of their funding, their after-school or summer school program has ended, and/or they have completed 40+ Guided Reading sessions. Occasionally, we have students several years in a row and these students are given a Visagraph test twice a school year.

In most cases, Visagraph pretests are given before students begin their Reading Plus program training. But there are several situations where we have to administer a Visagraph test shortly after beginning the program. This scenario usually happens when numerous students start on the same date; we just don't have the time to give everyone the Visagraph pre-assessment, so we have to schedule another time to complete this testing. On the other hand, the Visagraph post-tests are always done after the student has completed the Reading Plus training. At the post-assessment, students usually complete the Reading Placement Appraisal (Form B), even though it's a placement test and not a posttest, then do a Visagraph posttest. Sometimes we run out of time and the Visagraph post-test is done a few weeks later instead of immediately after.

Following are some typical samples of subjects' pretest and posttest reports.

In Figure 7.1, a grade three subject's pretest indicates:

- All FRP skills are well below grade three normative behaviors
- Reading Rate is only 57 words per minute with some rereading
- Grade Level Efficiency is only 1.0.

In Figure 7.2, the same grade three subject's posttest indicates:

- All FRP skills are now better than grade three norms
- Reading Rate is now 136 words per minute
- Grade Level Efficiency is now 4.1.

In Figure 7.3, a grade four subject's pretest indicates:

- A very high number of Fixations in relation to grade level four norms
- A very low Reading Rate of 88 words per minute in relation to grade level four norms
- A slightly high Directional Attack Difficulty of 18 percent
- Grade Level Efficiency is very low at 1.6.

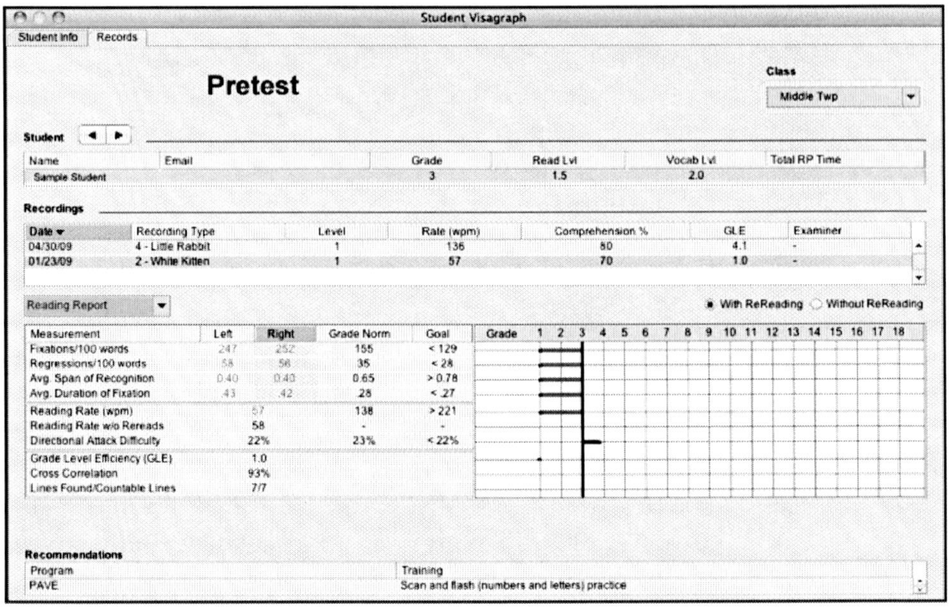

Figure 7.1

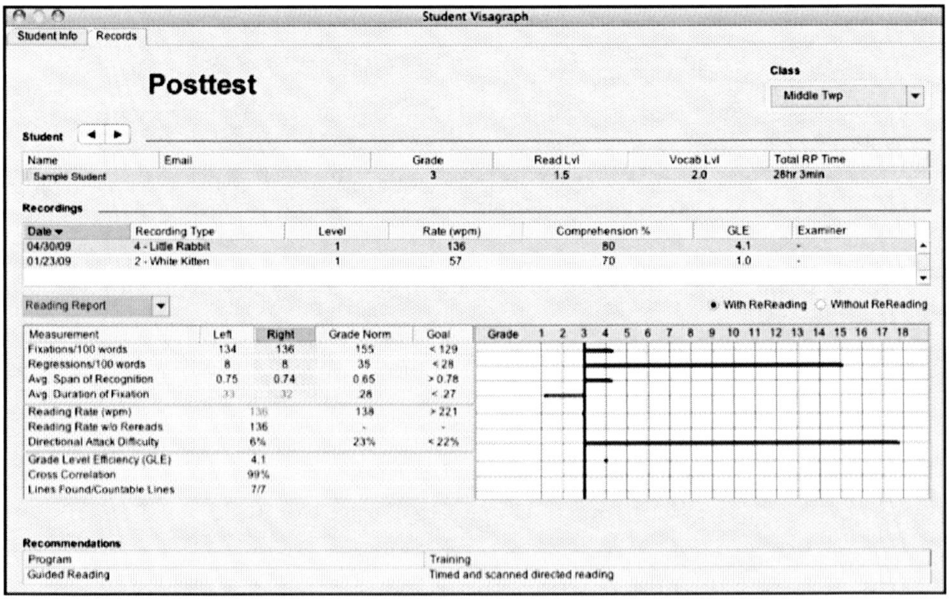

Figure 7.2

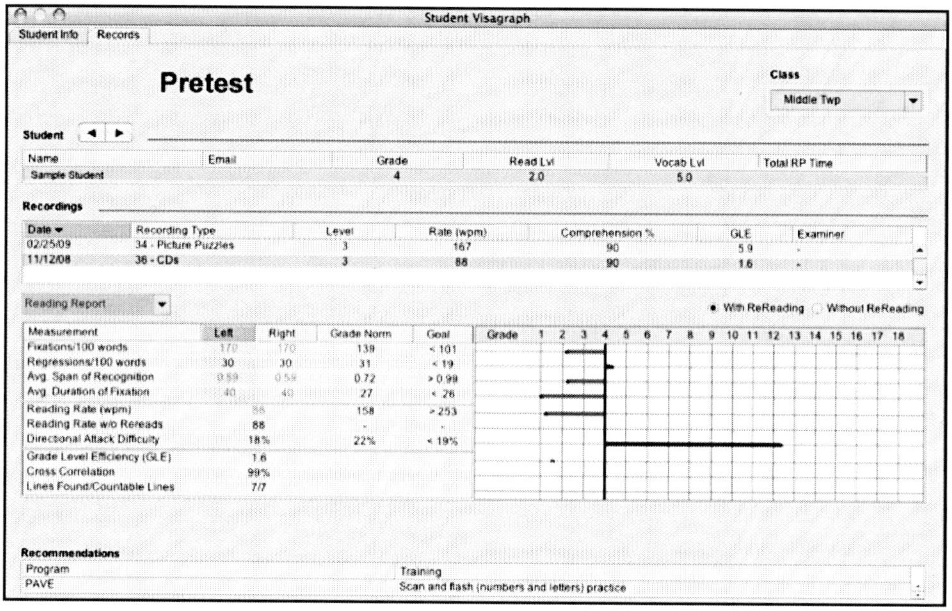

Figure 7.3

In Figure 7.4, the same grade four subject's posttest indicates:

- Most FRP skills are better than grade level four norms
- Reading Rate is higher than grade level norms at 167 words per minute
- Directional Attack Difficulty dropped to 8 percent
- Grade Level Efficiency is now 5.9.

In Figure 7.5, a grade four subject's pretest indicates:

- All FRP skills are well below grade level four norms
- Reading Rate is only 107 words per minute
- Grade Level Efficiency is only 1.2.

In Figure 7.6, the same grade four subject's posttest indicates:

- All FRP skills are now at or above grade level four norms
- Reading Rate is now 167 words per minute
- Grade Level Efficiency is now 5.6.

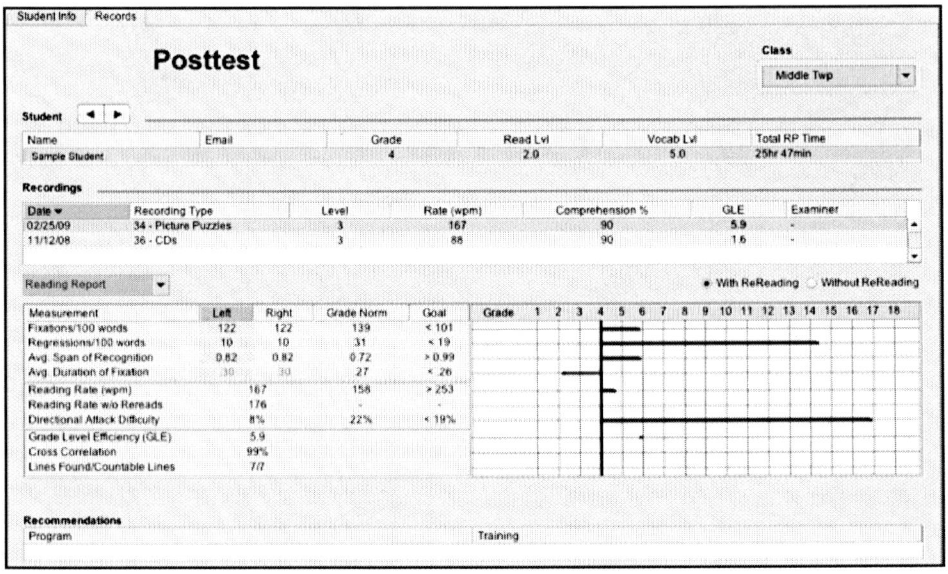

Figure 7.4

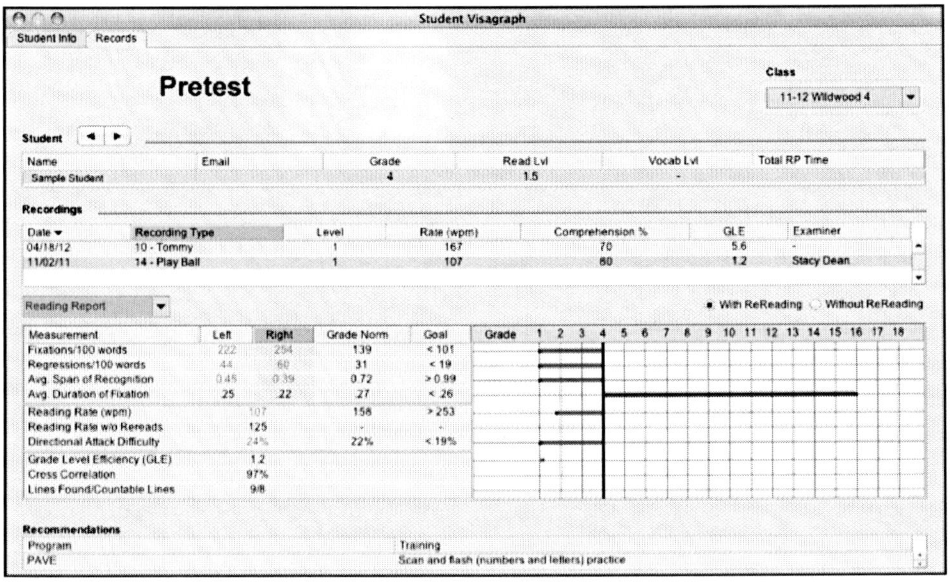

Figure 7.5

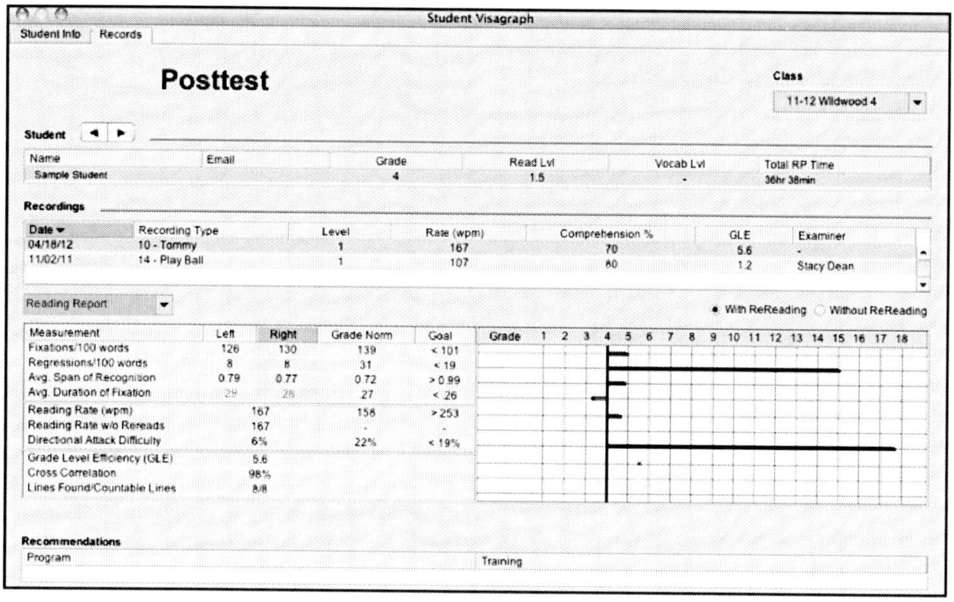

Figure 7.6

In Figure 7.7, a grade seven subject's pretest indicates:

- All FRP skills are well below grade level seven norms
- Reading Rate is 111 words per minute
- Grade Level Efficiency is only 1.5.

In Figure 7.8, the same grade seven subject's posttest indicates:

- FRP skills are close to grade level seven norms
- Reading Rate is 250 words per minute
- Grade Level Efficiency is now 10.1.

In Figure 7.9, a grade eight subject's pretest indicates:

- All FRP skills are well below grade level eight norms
- Reading Rate is only 111 words per minute
- Grade Level Efficiency is only 2.6.

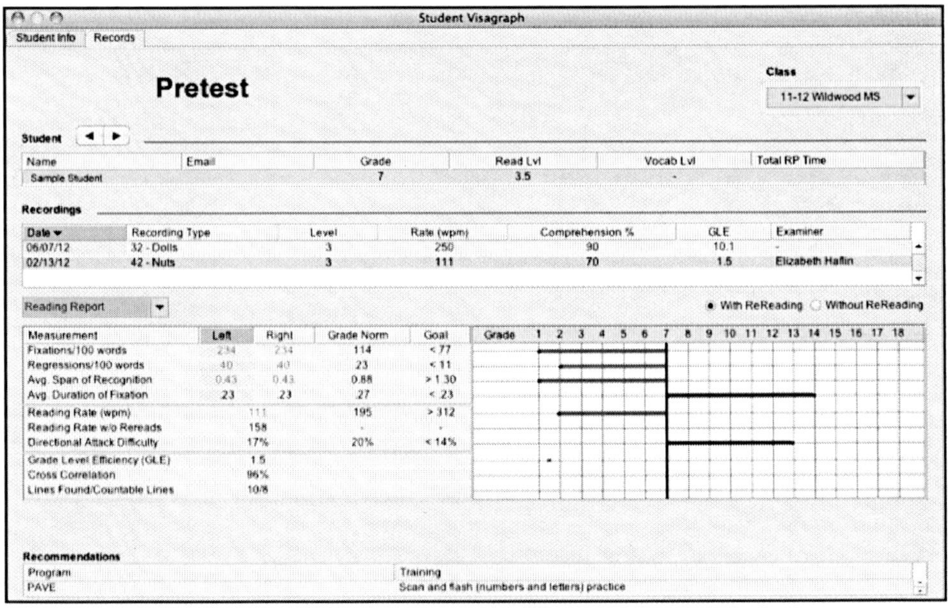

Figure 7.7

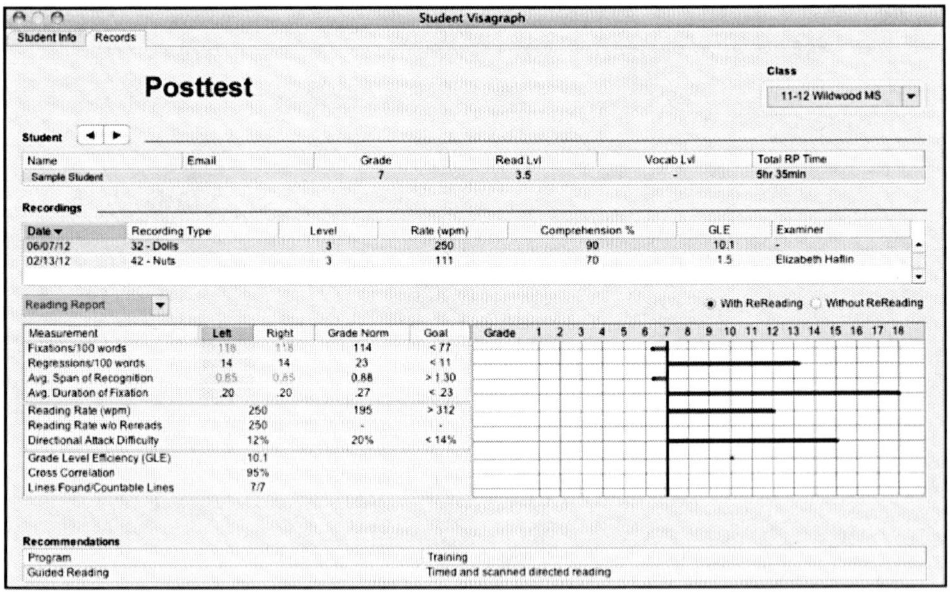

Figure 7.8

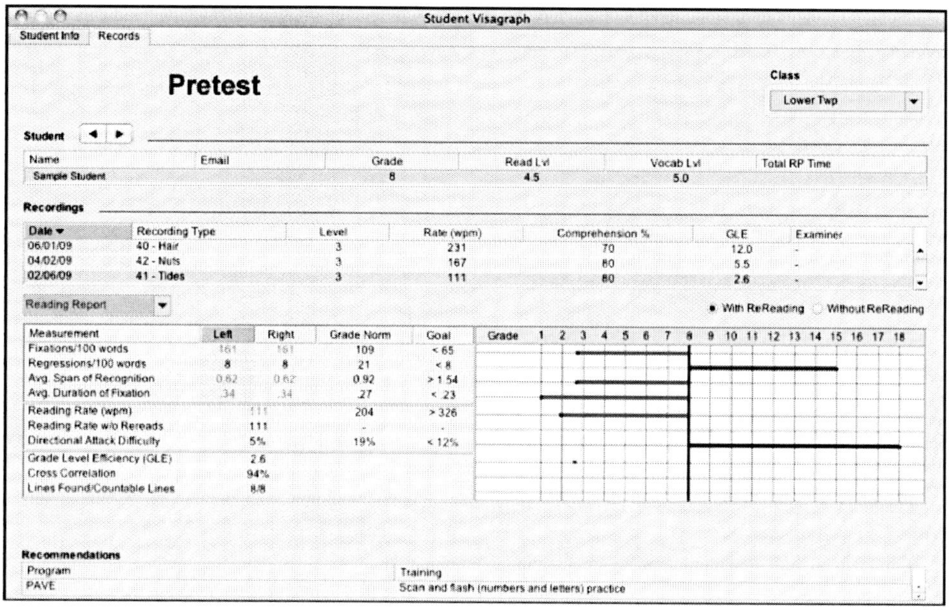

Figure 7.9

In Figure 7.10, the same grade eight subject's posttest indicates:

- All FRP skills are better than grade level eight norms

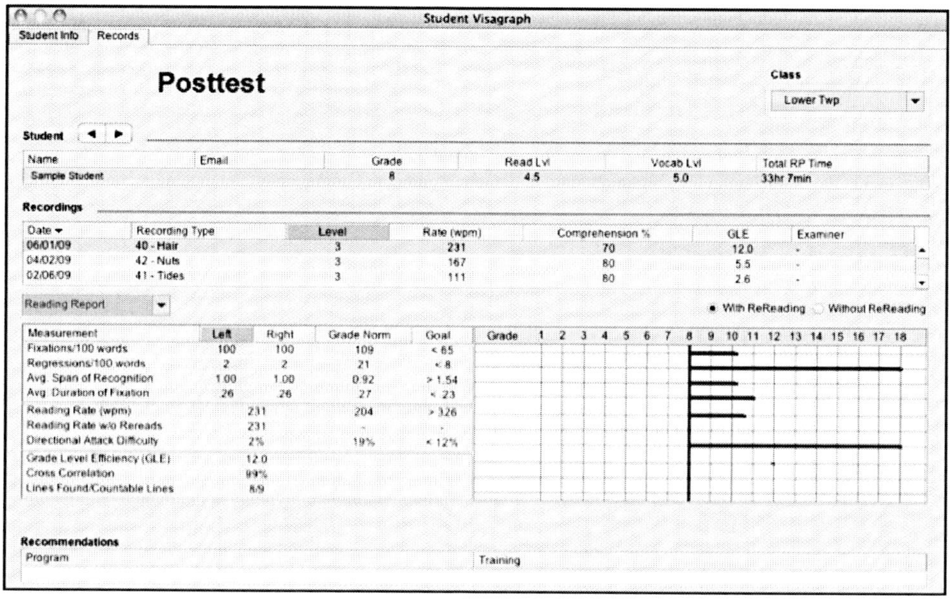

Figure 7.10

- Reading Rate is now 231 words per minute
- Grade Level Efficiency is now 12.0.

Tom Kroeger
Optimum Reading, LLC
Livonia, Michigan
248–471–8630
kroegert@optimumreading.com

With Optimum Reading, my typical program includes the use of Visagraph exams. As an incentive, I offer the 10-day Reading Plus trial along with a Visagraph exam before my clients begin their training program.

The 10-day trial and initial Visagraph testing serve as both a customer incentive and a screening opportunity for me. The Visagraph allows me to see if there is enough visual effectiveness to generate success. The trial period also gives me a sense of the student's willingness to complete lessons in a timely fashion.

The Visagraph testing has a number of benefits. First, clients are usually able to see there is a gap between their own skills and those of the normative group. Second, it provides me the ability to see if the student is likely to succeed with ReadingPlus. If there appear to be too many visual/functional problems, I may initially refer the client to vision therapy from a developmental optometrist. On occasion, I have had students score so highly that I was able to send the family off with the knowledge that their child is as exceptional as they had hoped.

Therefore I administer the Visagraph test with all initial clients and certainly after ReadingPlus use.

When the family chooses to proceed beyond the initial testing, the four-month trial begins. All the recommended clients for this project have been assigned to a class labeled "Success." Post-Visagraph tests are given near or after the training program expiration.

I recommend that students work in ReadingPlus three times per week, which can be done at home, and this allows them to be complete 50 to 60 lessons. Since these students typically work from home, life gets in the way of consistent effort in any given four-month period. Vacation, holidays, 4-H, school projects, and sports have all taken priority. Despite all that we see some very impressive improvements in visual/functional skills and reading efficiency in general. The pretest

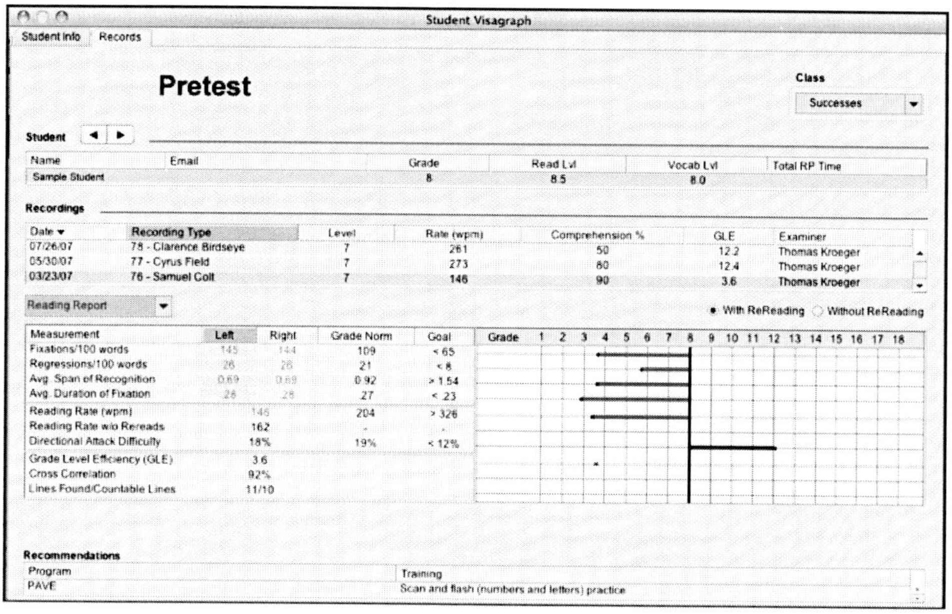

Figure 7.11

and posttest Visagraph reports indicate the relative degree of success we have experienced.

In Figure 7.11, a grade eight subject's pretest indicates:

- All FRP skills are lower than grade level eight norms
- Reading Rate is only 146 words per minute with some rereading
- Grade Level Efficiency is only 3.6.

In Figure 7.12, the same grade eight subject's posttest indicates:

- All FRP skills are better than grade level eight norms
- Reading Rate is now 273 words per minute with no rereading
- Grade Level Efficiency is now 12.4.

In Figure 7.13, a grade 10 subject's pretest indicates:

- Fixations are higher than grade level 10 norms
- Reading Rate is 158 words per minute
- Grade Level Efficiency is 3.9.

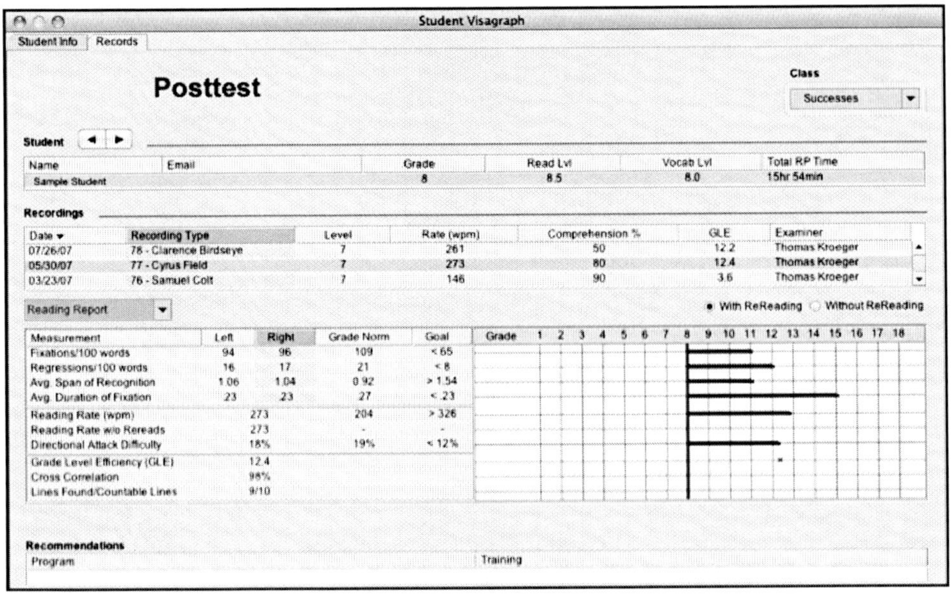

Figure 7.12

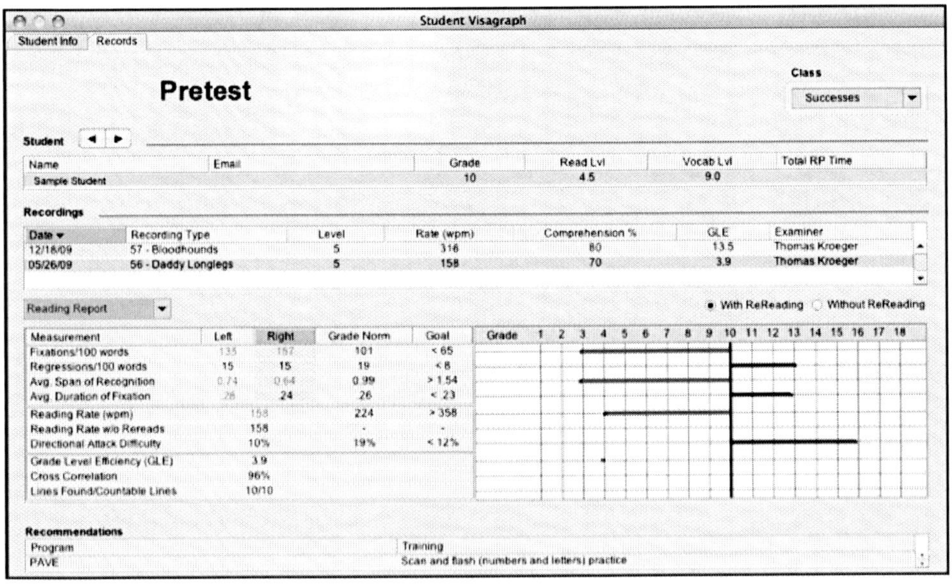

Figure 7.13

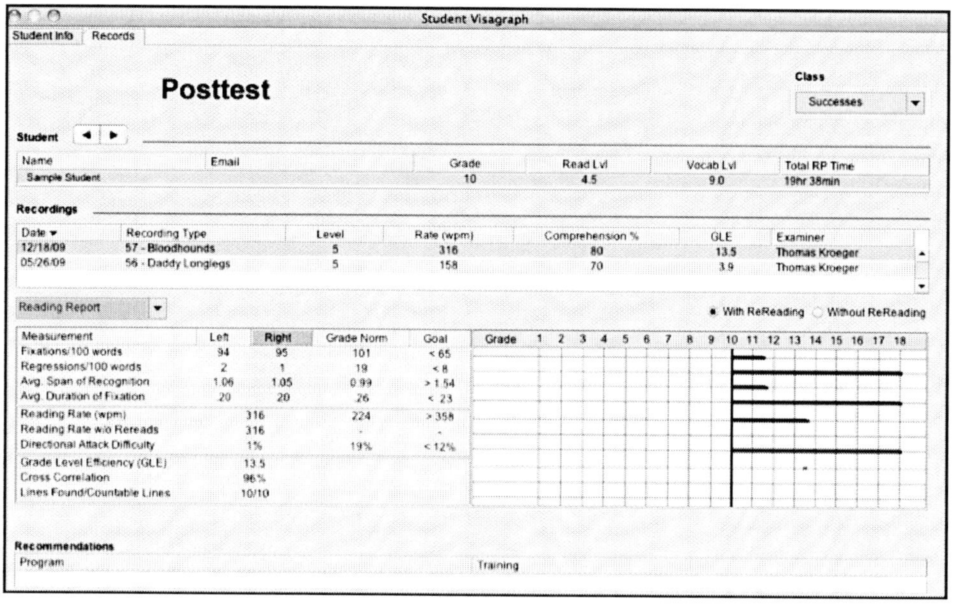

Figure 7.14

In Figure 7.14, the same grade 10 subject's posttest indicates:

- All FRP skills have improved
- Reading Rate is now 316 words per minute with no rereading
- Grade Level Efficiency is now 13.5.

In Figure 7.15, an adult subject's pretest indicates:

- All FRP skills are lower than expected for an adult
- Reading Rate is only 250 words per minute
- Grade Level Efficiency is 9.7.

In Figure 7.16, the same adult subject's posttest indicates:

- All FRP skills are better than expected in relation to adult norms
- Reading Rate is now 500 words per minute with no rereading
- Grade Level Efficiency is 16.9.

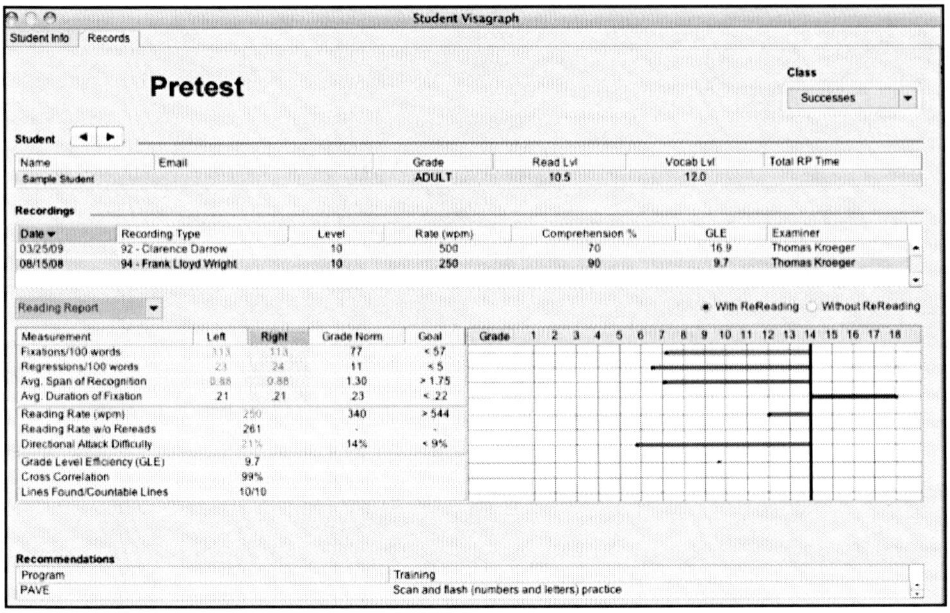

Figure 7.15

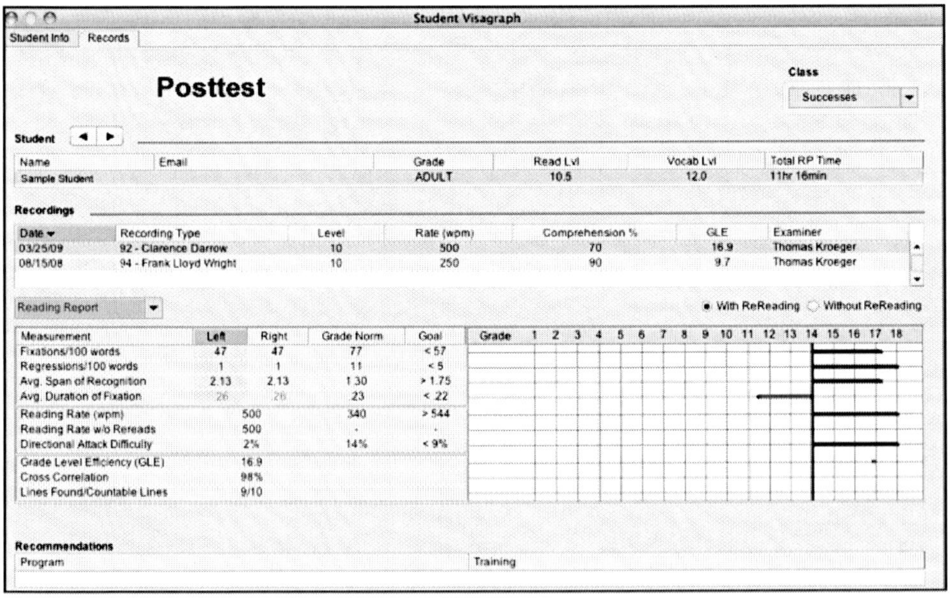

Figure 7.16

Megan Hudson, DC
Center Director
Brain Balance Achievement Center of West Springfield
West Springfield, Massachusetts 01089
413-737-5437
www.brainbalancecenters.com

I appreciate the opportunity to share my experience using the Visagraph, as I have found it to be a valuable assessment tool. In fact, I am delighted to share a few of my positive results with the hope that it will increase utilization of the device.

I have been using the Visagraph as an assessment tool for several years in two main settings and will briefly describe them each.

I currently own and operate a Brain Balance Achievement Center in West Springfield, Massachusetts. We are a supplemental education center (after school program) that works with children in grades K–12 who present with a wide range of learning and behavioral challenges. We see students who have been diagnosed with AD/HD, autism spectrum disorders (Asperger's, Pervasive Developmental Disorders-NOS, dyspraxia, dyslexia, OCD, ODD, Tourette's, Reactive Attachment Disorder, Central Auditory Processing Disorders, Learning Disabilities, Non-verbal Learning Disabilities). We also have students who are struggling, but not enough to qualify for a diagnosis or label.

We perform a comprehensive assessment to determine which brain hemisphere is functionally weaker in relation to the other, and then have the students participate in our 12-week program (36 one-hour sessions three times a week for 12 weeks) involving specific physical and academic exercises designed to strengthen the weaker hemisphere, thereby increasing the functional connectivity of the whole brain. This results in increased physical coordination, strength, and timing/rhythm, and increased academic performance and improvements in behavior and social skills. The assessment process involves a sensory motor component and an academic component. The results of the assessment determine candidacy for the program and also determine the curriculum for each student. There is also a nutritional component to the program in addition to home exercises.

When appropriate, we give the students a Visagraph test during the cognitive portion of the initial assessment and again during the post-program reassessment. I love to have the information the Visagraph provides. Sometimes I will use the visual skill assessment to measure students' fixations and saccades, and I wish that I could also use it to measure convergence and pursuits. The Brain Balance program is protocol driven and as all the centers are using the same protocols, we officially only use the Visagraph as a reading assessment tool.

Each student's program is individualized according to the various levels at which he or she tests initially and according to which side of the brain is being specifically addressed. Depending upon the result of the assessment, some of the students use Reading Plus as a part of their curriculum.

Before I opened this Brain Balance Center, I was practicing as a chiropractor focusing on Hemispheric Integration Therapy with kids and adults through the use of a Functional Neurology approach. I used the Visagraph as an assessment tool for a wide range of cases. Sometimes I used it before I did a treatment with a patient and then again immediately after to see what changed. Usually I would look at the visual skills. I did have a few patients who started using Reading Plus in conjunction with the clinical treatment I provided and the Visagraph was a great tool to measure efficacy of the combined approach.

Following are two examples of Visagraph pretest and posttest results. Figure 7.17 is a nine-year-old Brain Balance student who came in with no label, but struggles with social skills and poor bladder control. His initial reading comprehension score was 70 percent at his grade level of four, with a GLE of 10.1.

He did not do any sessions of Reading Plus. His right brain skills were addressed in the program. In Figure 7.18, his post-program assessment shows an increase in his GLE to 13.2 at a fifth grade level with 100 percent comprehension. In this case, the increased time of his Average Duration of Fixation is not seen as a decreased skill as the rest of his findings improved, including his comprehension at a higher grade level than his initial test. His bladder control improved significantly.

Figure 7.19 is of a 16-year-old Brain Balance student in tenth grade, with a label of Pervasive Developmental Disorder-NOS. He scored 70 percent in comprehension at a level 10 reading selection on his initial Visagraph test, with a GLE of 3.5.

After the 12-week Brain Balance program, the same student scored 80 percent comprehension at a level 7 reading selection, with a GLE of 12.2. He worked on his right brain and did Reading Plus five times

Reading Plus

Student:
Class: Brain Balance
Grade: 4
Examiner: Visagraph Administrator
Visagraph

Recording Type: 53 - Sign Language
Level: 4

Pretest

Reading Report 09/14/2011

Measurement	Left	Right	Grade Norm	Goal
Fixations/100 words	106	105	139	< 101
Regressions/100 words	12	12	31	< 19
Avg. Span of Recognition	0.94	0.95	0.72	> 0.99
Avg. Duration of Fixation	.25	.26	.27	< .26
Reading Rate (wpm)	222		158	> 253
Reading Rate w/o Rereads	231		-	-
Directional Attack Difficulty	11%		22%	< 19%
Grade Level Efficiency (GLE)	10.1			
Cross Correlation	95%			
Lines Found/ Countable Lines	9/11			

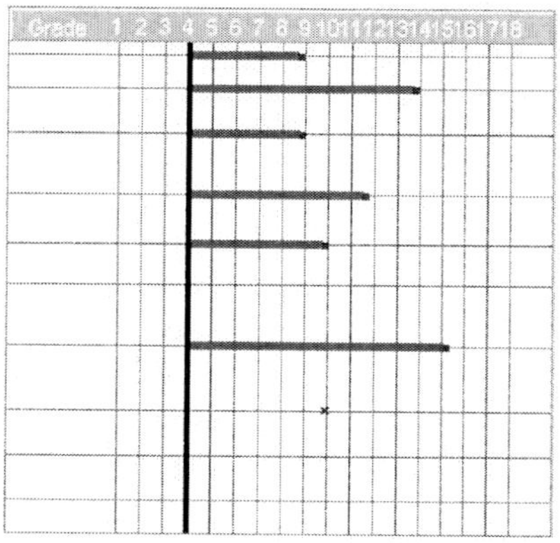

Figure 7.17

Reading Plus

Student:
Class: Brain Balance
Grade: 4
Examiner: Visagraph Administrator
Visagraph

Recording Type: 55 - Camels
Level: 5

Posttest

Reading Report 02/13/2012

Measurement	Left	Right	Grade Norm	Goal
Fixations/100 words	80	82	139	< 101
Regressions/100 words	8	8	31	< 19
Avg. Span of Recognition	1.25	1.22	0.72	> 0.99
Avg. Duration of Fixation	.29	.28	.27	< .26
Reading Rate (wpm)	261		158	> 253
Reading Rate w/o Rereads	273		-	-
Directional Attack Difficulty	10%		22%	< 19%
Grade Level Efficiency (GLE)	13.2			
Cross Correlation	98%			
Lines Found/ Countable Lines	9/10			

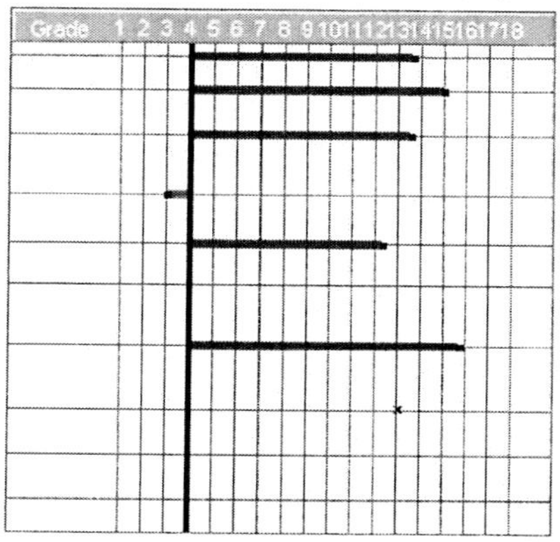

Figure 7.18

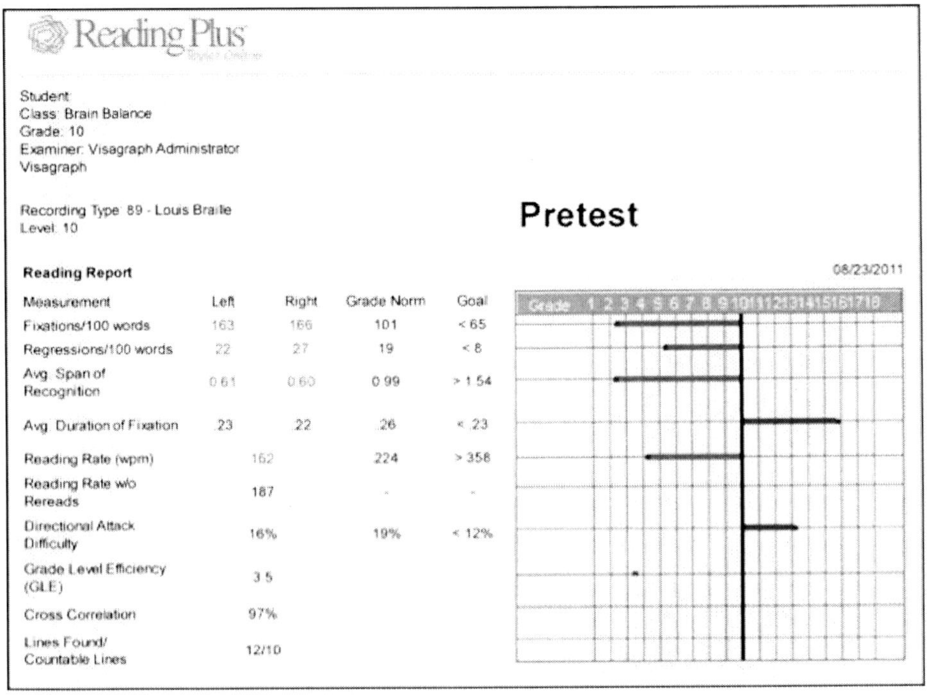

Reading Plus

Student
Class: Brain Balance
Grade: 10
Examiner: Visagraph Administrator
Visagraph

Recording Type: 89 - Louis Braille
Level: 10

Pretest

Reading Report 08/23/2011

Measurement	Left	Right	Grade Norm	Goal
Fixations/100 words	163	166	101	< 65
Regressions/100 words	22	27	19	< 8
Avg. Span of Recognition	0.61	0.60	0.99	> 1.54
Avg. Duration of Fixation	.23	.22	.26	< .23
Reading Rate (wpm)	162		224	> 358
Reading Rate w/o Rereads	187		-	-
Directional Attack Difficulty	16%		19%	< 12%
Grade Level Efficiency (GLE)	3.5			
Cross Correlation	97%			
Lines Found/ Countable Lines	12/10			

Figure 7.19

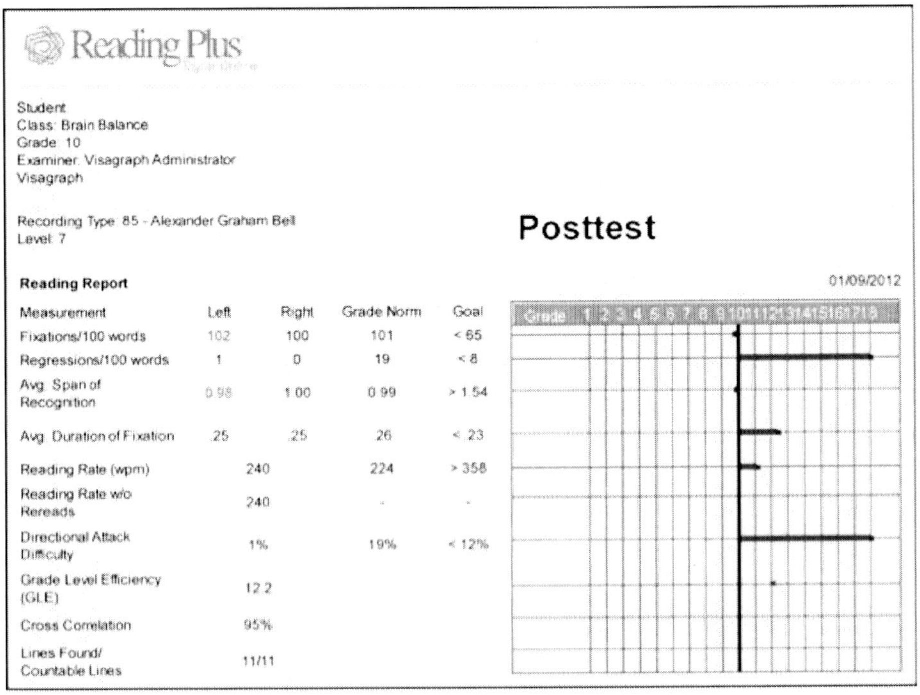

Reading Plus

Student
Class: Brain Balance
Grade: 10
Examiner: Visagraph Administrator
Visagraph

Recording Type: 85 - Alexander Graham Bell
Level: 7

Posttest

Reading Report 01/09/2012

Measurement	Left	Right	Grade Norm	Goal
Fixations/100 words	102	100	101	< 65
Regressions/100 words	1	0	19	< 8
Avg. Span of Recognition	0.98	1.00	0.99	> 1.54
Avg. Duration of Fixation	.25	.25	.26	< .23
Reading Rate (wpm)	240		224	> 358
Reading Rate w/o Rereads	240		-	-
Directional Attack Difficulty	1%		19%	< 12%
Grade Level Efficiency (GLE)	12.2			
Cross Correlation	95%			
Lines Found/ Countable Lines	11/11			

Figure 7.20

during the program. The changes, as seen in Figure 7.20, are due to increased efficiency in his ability to coordinate his eye movements, as well as selecting a reading passage that is more appropriate to his actual reading level.

3D Learner Inc.
Mira Halpert, M Ed
Boca Raton, Florida
561–361–7495
mire.halpert@gmail.com
success@3dlearner.com
www.3dlearner.com

We do Visagraph pretests and posttests on every student we see as part of our initial assessment. It has become an "ah ha" moment for the parents to realize that reading does in fact include eye-movement behavior when we show them the results of their child's Visagraph pre-training results. Also, after students look at their Simulation, they are convinced that their reading improvement is just a matter of skills and not their "smarts."

The pretest and posttest samples indicate the kinds of gains students have been able to achieve using Gemstone Foundation, 3D Learner Word Building Program, Visagraph skills training, and ReadingPlus. I would also like to mention that a number of our students have been introduced to ReadingPlus in their schools; therefore, some of the improvements result from school practice.

After only five weeks of reading training during a brief summer session, the Visagraph provided the ability to show parents the post Visagraph test results, which were amazing. Parents are stunned but appreciative to get an honest reading of their child's silent reading comprehension level. Although often low, they are delighted to realize that there is a way to significantly increase reading rate and comprehension over a four-month period. Following are some samples of pretest and posttest results.

In Figure 7.21, a grade seven subject's pretest indicates:

- FRP skills are lower than grade seven norms
- Reading Rate is only 94 words per minute
- Grade Level Efficiency is only 1.2.

Reading Plus

Student:
Class: USchool
Grade: 7
Examiner: Mira Halpert
3D Learner

Recording Type: 16 - Letters
Level: 2
Comprehension %: 100

Pretest

Reading Report 06/12/2012

Measurement	Left	Right	Grade Norm	Goal
Fixations/100 words	232	232	114	< 77
Regressions/100 words	52	54	23	< 11
Avg. Span of Recognition	0.43	0.43	0.88	> 1.30
Avg. Duration of Fixation	28	28	.27	< .23
Reading Rate (wpm)	94		195	> 312
Reading Rate w/o Rereads	130		-	-
Directional Attack Difficulty	23%		20%	< 14%
Grade Level Efficiency (GLE)	1.2			
Cross Correlation	95%			
Lines Found/ Countable Lines	11/7			

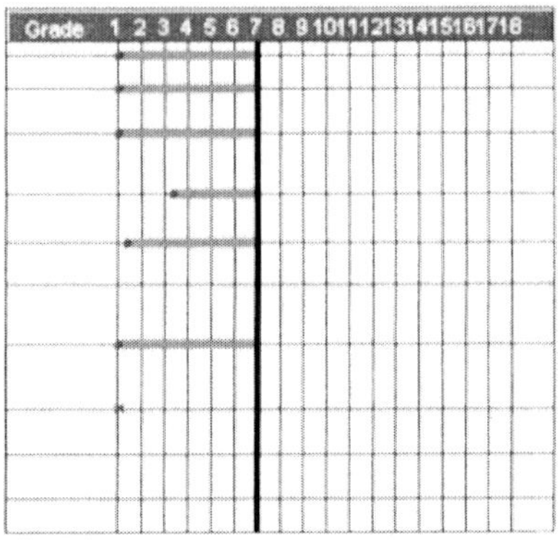

Figure 7.21

In Figure 7.22, the same grade seven subject's posttest indicates:

- FRP skills are better than grade nine level norms
- Reading Rate has improved to 273 words per minute with no rereading
- Grade Level Efficiency is now 10.5.

In Figure 7.23, a grade nine subject's pretest indicates:

- FRP skills are lower than grade nine norms
- Reading Rate is only 136 words per minute
- Grade Level Efficiency is only 3.5.

In Figure 7.24, the same grade nine subject's posttest indicates:

- FRP skills are better than grade nine level norms
- Reading Rate has improved to 182 words per minute with no rereading
- Grade Level Efficiency is now 9.1.

Reading Plus

Student:
Class: USchool
Grade: 7
Examiner: Mira Halpert
3D Learner

Recording Type: 15 - Firehouse
Level: 2
Comprehension %: 90

Posttest

Reading Report

07/11/2012

Measurement	Left	Right	Grade Norm	Goal
Fixations/100 words	88	98	114	< 77
Regressions/100 words	16	28	23	< 11
Avg. Span of Recognition	1.14	1.02	0.88	> 1.30
Avg. Duration of Fixation	.27	.24	.27	< .23
Reading Rate (wpm)	250		195	> 312
Reading Rate w/o Rereads	273		-	-
Directional Attack Difficulty	29%		20%	< 14%
Grade Level Efficiency (GLE)	10.5			
Cross Correlation	86%			
Lines Found/ Countable Lines	6/7			

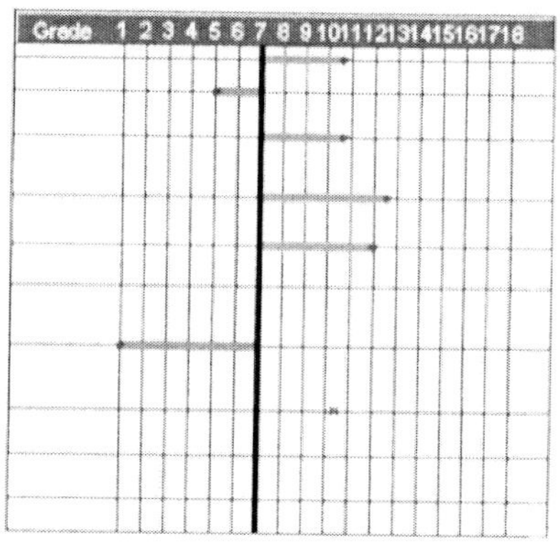

Figure 7.22

In Figure 7.25, a grade 10 subject's pretest indicates:

- FRP skills are lower than grade 10 norms
- Reading Rate is 200 words per minute
- Grade Level Efficiency is only 8.2.

In Figure 7.26, the same grade 10 subject's posttest indicates:

- FRP skills are better than grade 10 level norms
- Reading Rate has improved to 240 words per minute with no rereading
- Grade Level Efficiency is now 12.2.

In Figure 7.27, a grade 10 subject's pretest indicates:

- All FRP skills are lower than grade 10 norms
- Reading Rate is only 194 words per minute
- Grade Level Efficiency is only 6.2.

Reading Plus

Student:
Class: USchool
Grade: 9
Examiner: Mira Halpert
3D Learner

Recording Type: 29 - Stamps
Level: 3
Comprehension %: 70

Pretest

Reading Report

06/12/2012

Measurement	Left	Right	Grade Norm	Goal
Fixations/100 words	141	138	105	< 65
Regressions/100 words	21	19	20	< 8
Avg. Span of Recognition	0.71	0.72	0.95	> 1.54
Avg. Duration of Fixation	31	32	.27	< .23
Reading Rate (wpm)	136		214	> 342
Reading Rate w/o Rereads	143		-	-
Directional Attack Difficulty	15%		19%	< 12%
Grade Level Efficiency (GLE)	3.5			
Cross Correlation	97%			
Lines Found/ Countable Lines	7/7			

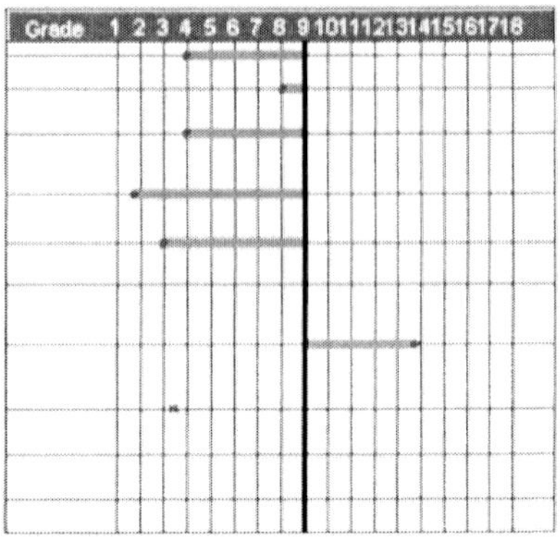

Figure 7.23

Reading Plus

Student:
Class: USchool
Grade: 9
Examiner: Mira Halpert
3D Learner

Recording Type: 56 - Daddy Longlegs
Level: 5
Comprehension %: 100

Posttest

Reading Report

07/11/2012

Measurement	Left	Right	Grade Norm	Goal
Fixations/100 words	98	98	105	< 65
Regressions/100 words	6	7	20	< 8
Avg. Span of Recognition	1.02	1.02	0.95	> 1.54
Avg. Duration of Fixation	34	34	.27	< .23
Reading Rate (wpm)	182		214	> 342
Reading Rate w/o Rereads	182		-	-
Directional Attack Difficulty	7%		19%	< 12%
Grade Level Efficiency (GLE)	9.1			
Cross Correlation	97%			
Lines Found/ Countable Lines	10/10			

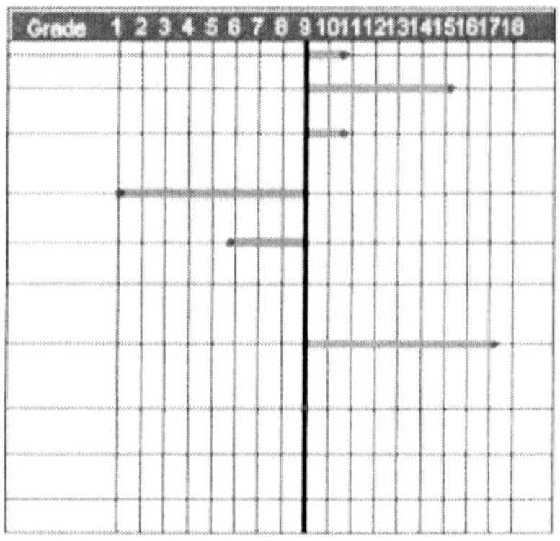

Figure 7.24

Reading Plus

Student:
Class: USchool
Grade: 10
Examiner: Mira Halpert
3D Learner

Recording Type: 44 - Corn
Level: 4
Comprehension %: 70

Pretest

Reading Report

06/12/2012

Measurement	Left	Right	Grade Norm	Goal
Fixations/100 words	115	117	101	< 65
Regressions/100 words	6	7	19	< 8
Avg. Span of Recognition	0.87	0.85	0.99	> 1.54
Avg. Duration of Fixation	.26	.26	.26	< .23
Reading Rate (wpm)	200		224	> 358
Reading Rate w/o Rereads	231		-	-
Directional Attack Difficulty	6%		19%	< 12%
Grade Level Efficiency (GLE)	8.2			
Cross Correlation	98%			
Lines Found/ Countable Lines	11/10			

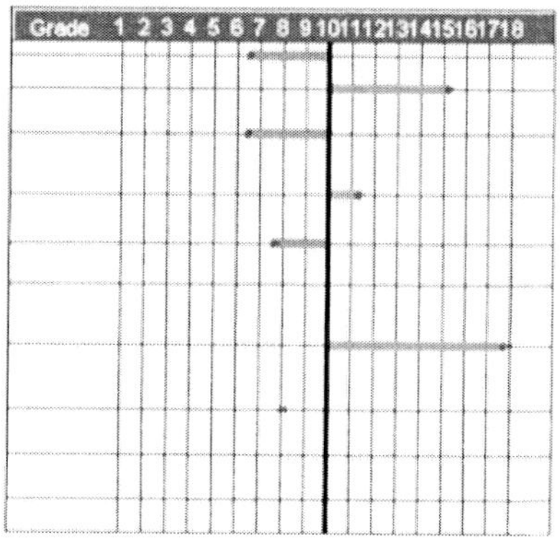

Figure 7.25

Reading Plus

Student:
Class: USchool
Grade: 10
Examiner: Mira Halpert
3D Learner

Recording Type: 76 - Samuel Colt
Level: 7
Comprehension %: 90

Posttest

Reading Report

07/11/2012

Measurement	Left	Right	Grade Norm	Goal
Fixations/100 words	98	99	101	< 65
Regressions/100 words	3	5	19	< 8
Avg. Span of Recognition	1.02	1.01	0.99	> 1.54
Avg. Duration of Fixation	.26	.25	.26	< .23
Reading Rate (wpm)	240		224	> 358
Reading Rate w/o Rereads	240		-	-
Directional Attack Difficulty	5%		19%	< 12%
Grade Level Efficiency (GLE)	12.2			
Cross Correlation	93%			
Lines Found/ Countable Lines	10/10			

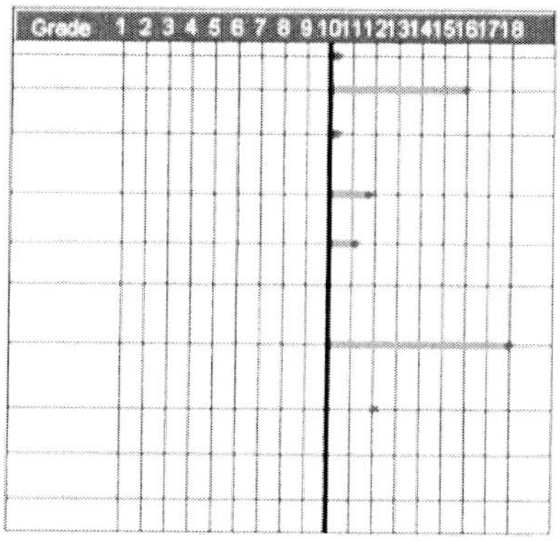

Figure 7.26

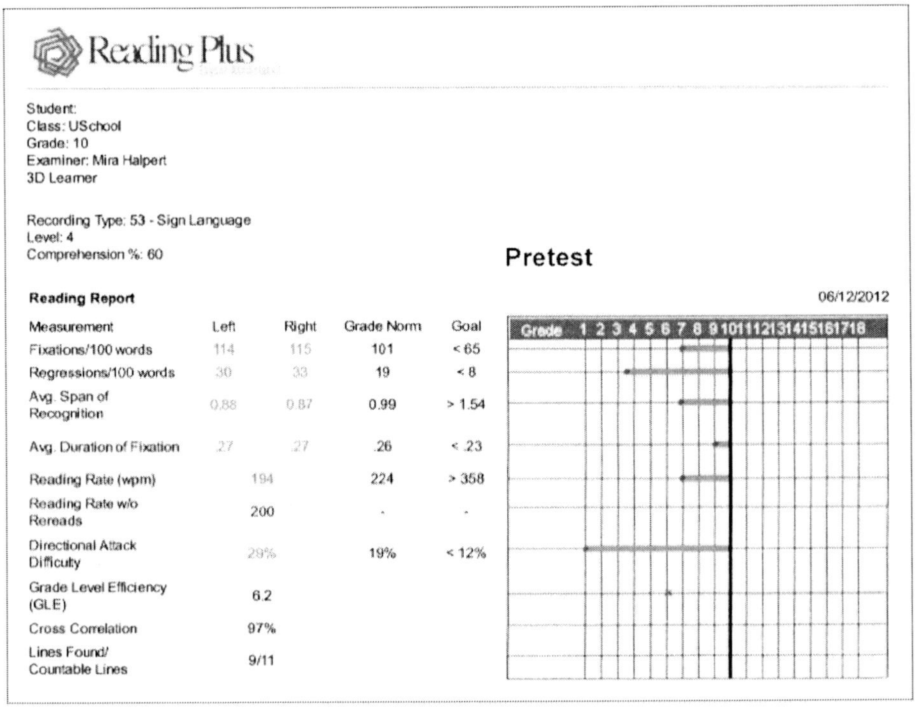

Reading Plus

Student:
Class: USchool
Grade: 10
Examiner: Mira Halpert
3D Learner

Recording Type: 53 - Sign Language
Level: 4
Comprehension %: 60

Pretest

Reading Report 06/12/2012

Measurement	Left	Right	Grade Norm	Goal
Fixations/100 words	114	115	101	< 65
Regressions/100 words	30	33	19	< 8
Avg. Span of Recognition	0.88	0.87	0.99	> 1.54
Avg. Duration of Fixation	.27	.27	.26	< .23
Reading Rate (wpm)	194		224	> 358
Reading Rate w/o Rereads	200		-	-
Directional Attack Difficulty	29%		19%	< 12%
Grade Level Efficiency (GLE)	6.2			
Cross Correlation	97%			
Lines Found/ Countable Lines	9/11			

Figure 7.27

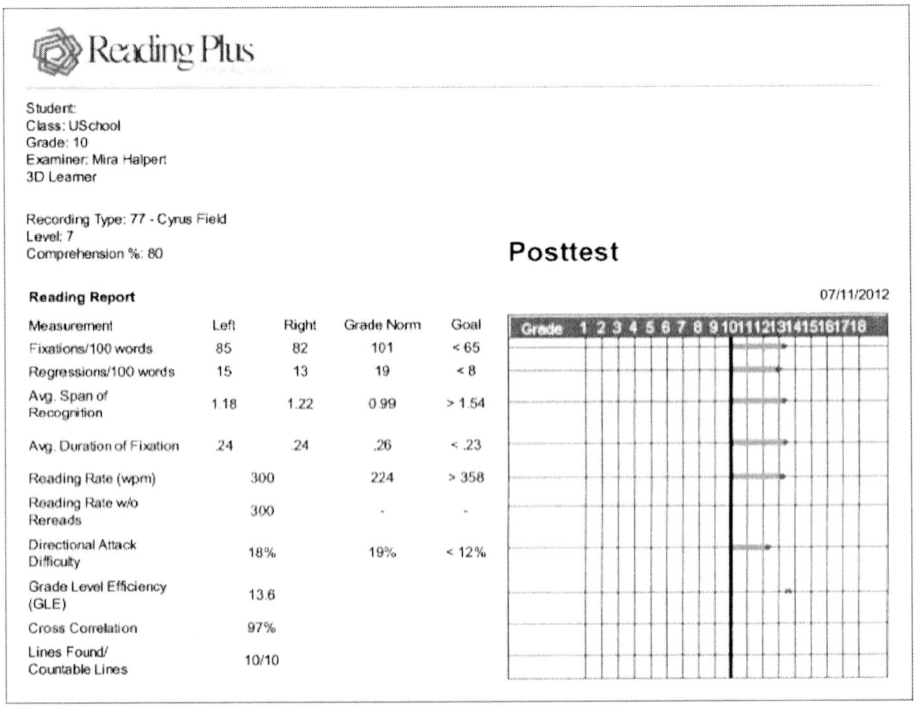

Reading Plus

Student:
Class: USchool
Grade: 10
Examiner: Mira Halpert
3D Learner

Recording Type: 77 - Cyrus Field
Level: 7
Comprehension %: 80

Posttest

Reading Report 07/11/2012

Measurement	Left	Right	Grade Norm	Goal
Fixations/100 words	85	82	101	< 65
Regressions/100 words	15	13	19	< 8
Avg. Span of Recognition	1.18	1.22	0.99	> 1.54
Avg. Duration of Fixation	.24	.24	.26	< .23
Reading Rate (wpm)	300		224	> 358
Reading Rate w/o Rereads	300		-	-
Directional Attack Difficulty	18%		19%	< 12%
Grade Level Efficiency (GLE)	13.6			
Cross Correlation	97%			
Lines Found/ Countable Lines	10/10			

Figure 7.28

In Figure 7.28, the same grade 10 subject's posttest indicates:

- FRP skills are better than grade 10 level norms
- Reading Rate is now 300 words per minute with no rereading
- Grade Level Efficiency is now 13.6.

Pat Rosenbury
Brainlinking, Inc.
Sandy, Utah
801–467–6278
info@brainlinking.com
www.brainlinking.com

In addition to the Reading Plus fluency-development program, during each four-month BrainLinking program, we also provide memory development, vision therapy, sensory integration, and concentration and focusing training.

We use the Visagraph with all of our BrainLinking clients prior to the beginning of their training programs, as well as four months later at the end of their programs. These Visagraph pretests and posttests enable us to provide definitive and authoritative printed reports for parents. In addition, we provide a written interpretation of the Visagraph results.

The pretest and posttest samples that follow are indicative of the overall improvements experienced by our clients.

In Figure 7.29, a grade four subject's pretest norms indicate close to grade level or above:

- Some FRP skills are lower than grade four norms
- Reading Rate is 167 words per minute (slightly higher than norms)
- Grade Level Efficiency is 4.2.

In Figure 7.30, the same grade four subject's posttest indicates:

- All FRP skills are remarkably better than grade four level norms
- Reading Rate is now 231 words per minute with no rereading
- Grade Level Efficiency is now well above grade at 11.1.

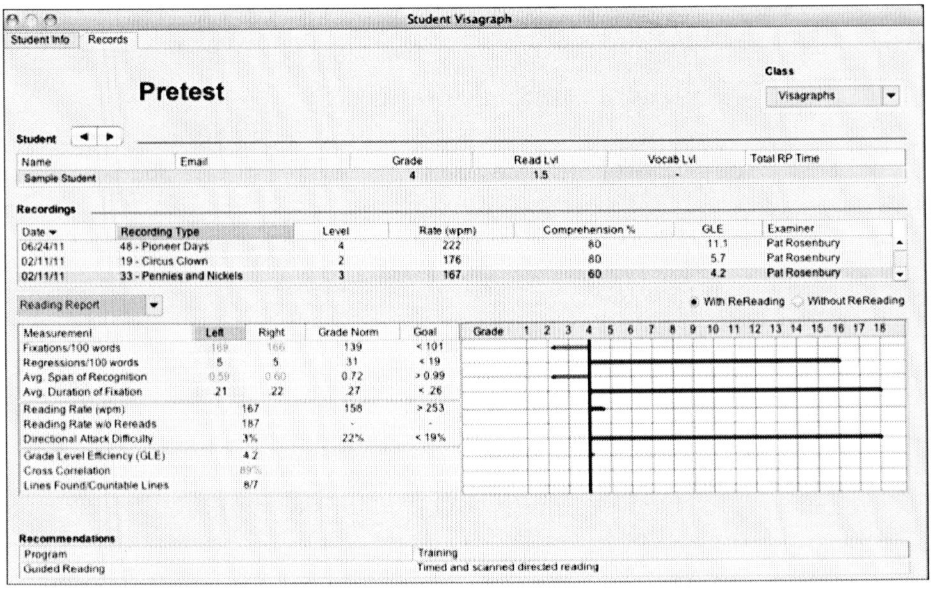

Figure 7.29

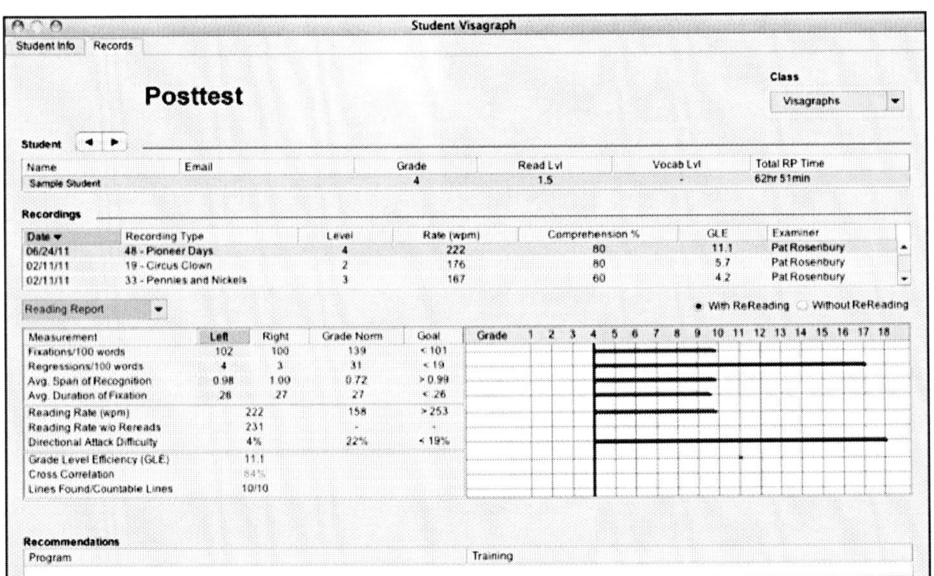

Figure 7.30

In Figure 7.31, a grade four subject's pretest indicates:

- FRP skills are lower than grade four norms
- Reading Rate is 97 words per minute
- Grade Level Efficiency is 1.7.

In Figure 7.32, the same grade four subject's posttest indicates:

- FRP skills are better than grade four level norms
- Reading Rate is now 140 words per minute
- Grade Level Efficiency is now 4.6.

In Figure 7.33, a grade five subject's pretest indicates:

- FRP skills are much lower than grade five norms
- Reading Rate is 130 words per minute
- Grade Level Efficiency is only 2.6.

In Figure 7.34, the same grade five subject's posttest indicates:

- FRP skills are remarkably better than grade five level norms
- Reading Rate is now 316 words per minute without rereading
- Grade Level Efficiency is now 14.3.

In Figure 7.35, a college level subject's pretest indicates:

- FRP skills are much lower than college level norms
- Reading Rate is 115 words per minute
- Grade Level Efficiency is only 2.6.

In Figure 7.36, the same college level subject's posttest indicates:

- FRP skills are improved to college level norms
- Reading Rate is now 316 words per minute without rereading
- Grade Level Efficiency is now 13.6.

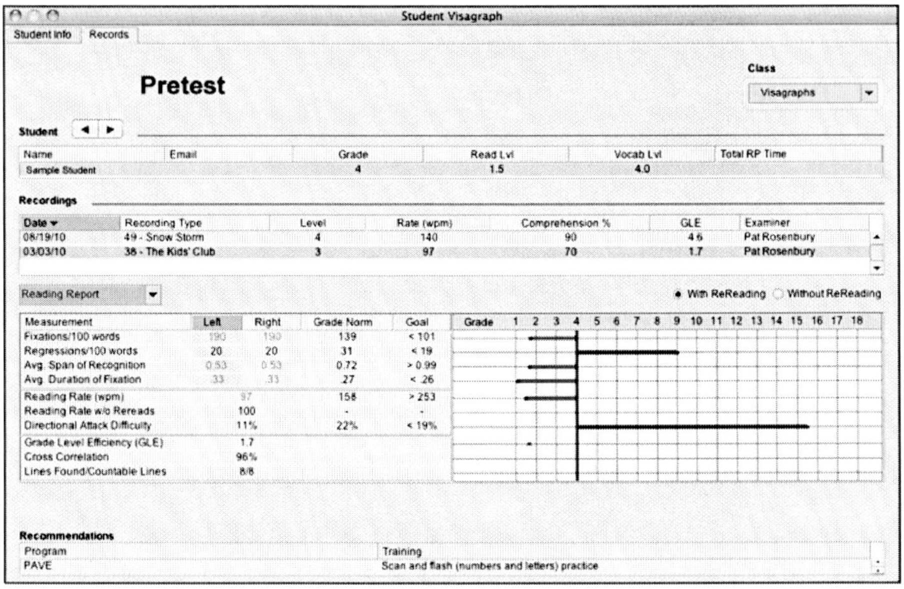

Figure 7.31

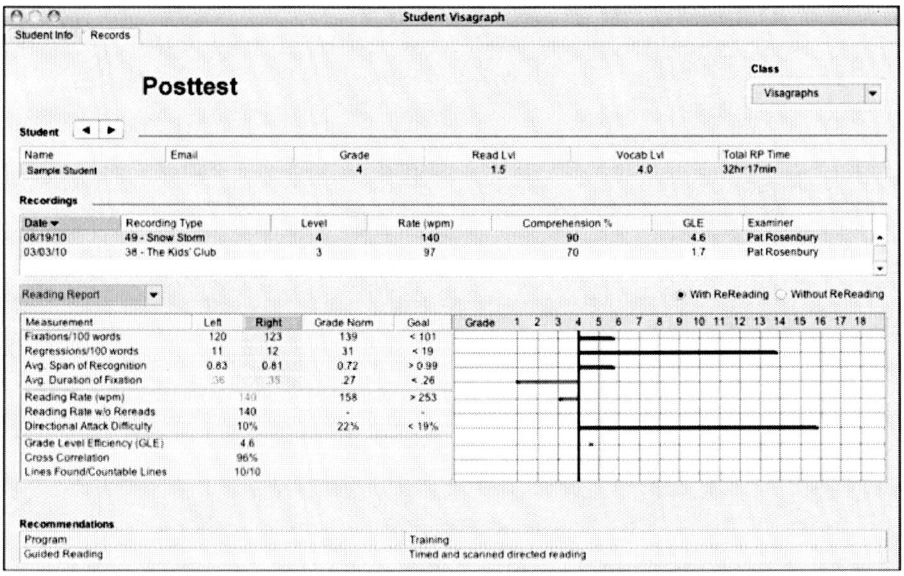

Figure 7.32

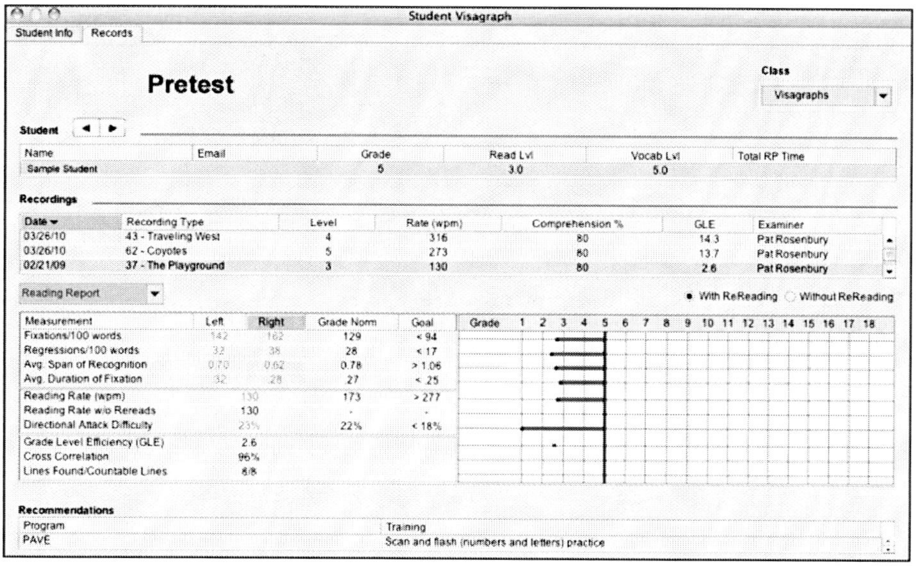

Figure 7.33

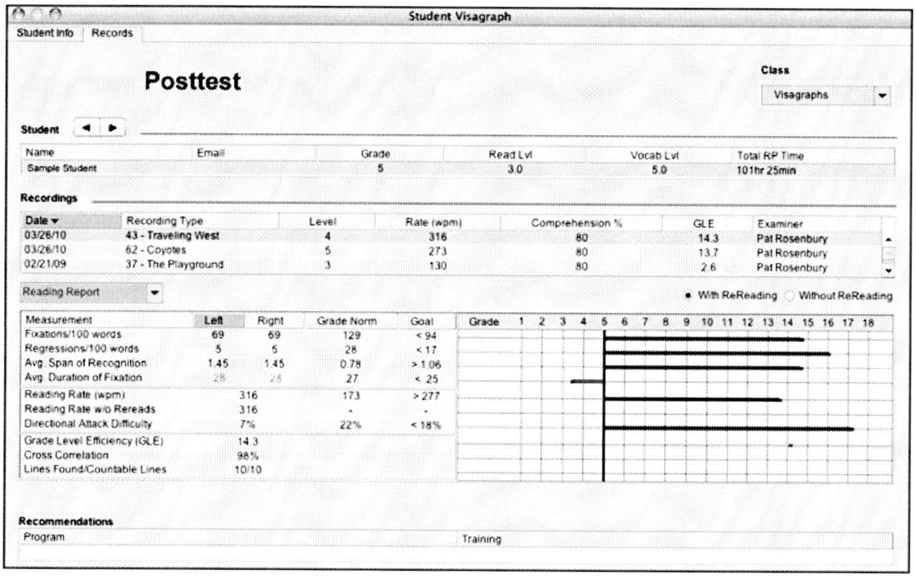

Figure 7.34

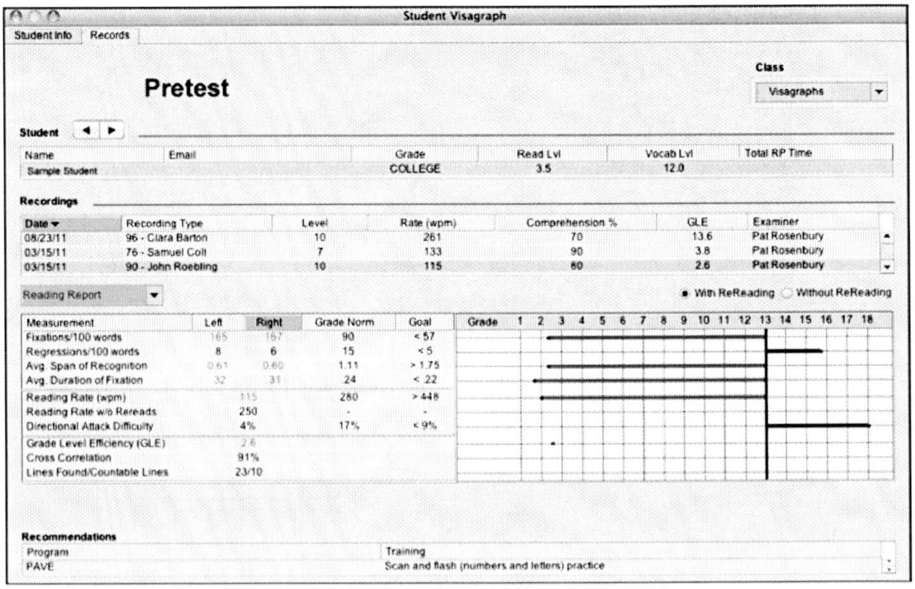

Figure 7.35

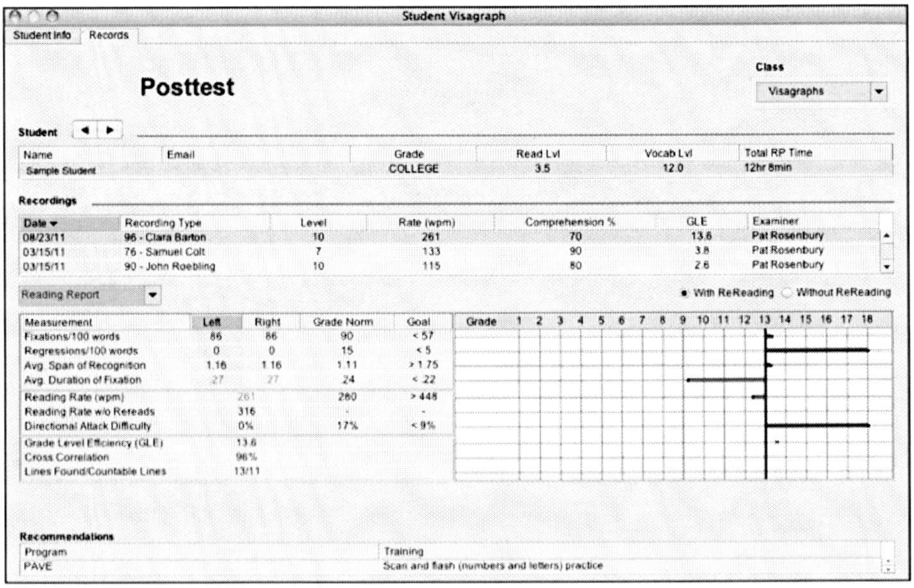

Figure 7.36

QUESTIONS THAT COULD ARISE AFTER READING THIS CHAPTER

1. How will you determine which of your clients require Visagraph testing?
2. How often should your clinic attendees be retested with the Visagraph?
3. How might Visagraph findings influence your use of today's web-based silent reading fluency-development programs?
4. How might the web-based fluency-development programs be employed in the home as well as in your clinic?
5. How might the Visagraph findings suggest a need for a follow-up fluency-development practice program at a later date?

Chapter 8

VISAGRAPH FIELD USE–VISION SPECIALISTS

Hundreds of optometrists use the Visagraph as part of their reading evaluation and visual/functional assessment. The use of the Visagraph will naturally vary considerably based on the optometrist's goals.

Leonard J. Press, OD, FCOVD, FAAO
Optometric Director, The Vision & Learning Center
Fair Lawn, New Jersey
www.pressvision.com

Clinical Insights into the Visagraph

In our Vision & Learning Center, the Visagraph has become an indispensable tool in the assessment of eye movements during silent reading. Due to the nature of our clinical population, the majority of whom have difficulties with the visual components of reading, we discovered at the outset that many of the poor readers exhibited considerable variability in their Visagraph Profiles.

After experimenting with several different protocols, we settled on an approach that gave us the most consistent results. We present the initial reading passage at two text levels below the patient's current grade placement. If either the comprehension score is below 70 percent, or the grade level equivalent (GLE) is below the child's current grade placement, we administer the second passage at a lower text level. The number of text levels we drop depends on the child's grade placement and consideration of both the comprehension score and the

GLE result. We will illustrate this with a couple of examples:

Example 1: The child is in fourth grade, therefore, Text Level 2 is selected.

Scenario 1

Passage 1 Result: GLE = 3.1 and Comprehension = 80 percent.

Decision: Administer Passage 2 at Text Level 1

Passage 2 Result: GLE = 4.5 and Comprehension = 100 percent

Scenario 2

Passage 1 Result: GLE = 5.8 and Comprehension = 50 percent

Decision: Administer Passage 2 at Text Level 1

Passage 2 Result: GLE = 4.5 and Comprehension = 100 percent

Discussion

Even though comprehension was good in Scenario 1, GLE was below grade level placement. Bear in mind that the questions asked are true/false, and the child has a 50 percent chance of guessing correctly even if the passage was not read. In both scenarios, Text Level 1 reflects a passage with a sight word vocabulary for which this child can execute an eye movement pattern commensurate with other children in the same grade who are achieving readers. This enables us to estimate that in both scenarios the child's GLE is approximately three grade levels below where it should be.

Example 2: The child is in eighth grade, therefore, Text Level 6 is selected.

Scenario 1

Passage 1 Result: GLE = 2.2 and Comprehension = 50 percent.

Decision: Administer Passage 2 at Text Level 3

Passage 2 Result: GLE = 2.5 and Comprehension = 80 percent

Decision: Administer Passage 3 at Text Level 1

Passage 3 Result: GLE = 2.9 and Comprehension = 90 percent

Scenario 2

Passage 1 Result: GLE = 10.1 and Comprehension = 90 percent

Decision: Administer Passage 2 at Text Level 8

Passage 2 Result: GLE = 6.4 and Comprehension = 80 percent

Discussion

When the child is older and in a higher grade placement, there is more latitude to drop down to passages considerably below grade level. In scenario 1, the child's GLE remains well below grade level irrespective of the Text Level selected. This is either a child with a fundamental ocular motor deficit, or a child who struggles with comprehension so that fluency is constrained by a slow or regressive scan path. In Scenario 2, passage 1 results were sufficiently strong in both GLE and comprehension to warrant going up two text levels. This proved to be too difficult and although comprehension was good, GLE was below grade level placement.

In a busy clinical setting, it is important to have protocols. Our colleagues at the SUNY College of Optometry, where I formerly served as Chief of the Vision Therapy Service, suggested baseline analyses and procedural guidelines that are similar to the protocols we use in practice. Ciuffreda, Ciuffreda, and Santos (2003) stressed the importance of administering multiple passages in order to derive a stable baseline against which the results of subsequent measures can be compared. Generally speaking the younger the child or the more hyperactivity the patient generates, the more variability there will be from one recording to the next due to excessive movement of the head and sensors.

Tannen and Ciuffreda (2007) proposed an addition to this protocol that is most useful for older children and adults. When the patient struggles with the first two passages, with GLE well below grade level placement on both, they administer a third passage at Text Level 1. The GLE of the third passage helps differentiate between two categories of patients:

Category 1: A patient who does not improve his or her GLE at least three grade levels above the GLE of either of the preceding two passages suggests an ocular motor efficiency problem.

Category 2: A patient who does improve his or her GLE at least three grade levels above the GLE of either of the preceding two passages. This suggests a language-based problem.

Although this is a very good generalization there will be some exceptions to the rule. Aside from the sight word vocabulary becoming easier with lower text levels, another feature is that the letters are larger in size and the inter-letter spacing increases. There are a subset of patients who will perform better at lower text levels not principally because of a language factor, but because they are sensitive to a visual crowding phenomenon as stated in the Eide Neurolearning Blog (2012). A form of sensory overload, crowding can be addressed by photo-enlarging print size in reading development practice, either by obtaining a larger print text of the same material, or using a Kindle or similar electronic reading devices to photo-enlarge text that is appropriate for the individual's sight word vocabulary. The improvement in ocular motor efficiency in this instance should directly aid reading fluency, and complements the scaffolding process built into the Reading Plus system.

Although the GLE is valuable as a weighted factor analysis of the composite variables being measured, there are nuances to be gained by inspecting the individual variables. It is normal for good readers to exhibit a 15 percent regression rate when eye movements are recorded during silent reading. Therefore an individual who shows a Regressions/100 words score that is at a grade level well above their actual grade's average is not necessarily being efficient.

We administer the Visagraph routinely to every child who presents for a sensorimotor evaluation. This is because the eye-movement recordings give us a level of objective information about eye movement accuracy that is not readily available though other testing. Occasionally we encounter a child whose parents did not report any concerns about reading on the initial intake or on our patient history checklist. In these instances, we administer the first passage at a Text Level equivalent to the child's actual grade placement in school, or their Grade Level Reading Performance as available through prior standardized testing. Nevertheless, the Visagraph may show a reduced GLE. When GLE is poor on passage one, we drop two Text Levels below for the second passage, and follow the same lines of analysis noted above. In some instances, it was a matter of text anxiety, and the child does better on the second passage at the same grade level. In other instances, the GLE is equally poor on the second passage at the same Text Level, and the child is struggling with reading to a greater extent than the parent suspects, and that is one reason why schoolwork takes so long to complete.

The Cross Correlation is considered a measure of how well the two eyes track in tandem. When the patient has instability or inefficiency in binocular vision, it is not uncommon to see performance deteriorate with each subsequent passage during a given recording session. One would expect under normal circumstances that if a child were given two reading passages at the same Text Level, the second passage would result in a GLE higher than the first passage. This is because there is a practice or learning effect from having knowledge of what the task is like. If the second passage has a GLE lower than the first passage, the most likely explanations for this are:

1. Loss of interest or attention
2. Testing fatigue
3. Pre-familiarity with subject matter of the higher Text Level passage

In our practice, we not only utilize the Visagraph to document reading performance prior to prescribing optometric vision therapy, but to compare reading performance with and without contemplated lens prescriptions. An individual may be noted to improve performance significantly by being prescribed glasses, by having the lens prescription changed, by having prism incorporated, or by optometric vision therapy.

When a program of optometric vision therapy is prescribed, obtaining consistent baseline Visagraph recordings becomes even more important. We utilize these recordings to compare changes when Visagraph testing is readministered during monthly progress evaluations. The Visagraph is a crucial part of our baseline data, which is used to objectively document progress and to help guide and refine the course of therapy. We also repeat Visagraph recordings when the patient is seen for subsequent progress evaluations after completion of the vision therapy program.

Thus far we have focused on the quantitative data available through the recordings, but there is valuable qualitative data as well. Most revealing is the Simulation option, which shows the combined effect of both eyes into a single scan path illustrated by a cursor. The playback can show the extent of regressions, erratic eye movements, and loss of place. One of the first times we used the Simulation, I noted that the cursor would go to the end of the line, drop down to the next line toward the right margin, backtrack toward the beginning of the line, and then proceed leftward toward the end of the line. The child was old enough to participate in the conference with the parents, during which we reviewed the Visagraph data together. I asked the student if there was awareness of doing this during reading. The student replied, "Sure. If I try to read normally, I get lost going from the end of one line to the beginning of the next one. This way if I drop down at the end of the line, it's easier to find the next line."

A common suggestion given by teachers to children who lose their place when reading is to use a window cutout or straight edge as a guide when reading. This is the approach used in the Reading Plus Guided Reading program, which employs a guided slot to expose words in a sequential left to right manner. It is obvious that the Visagraph is an important objective tool that can help assess the effectiveness of a Reading Plus intervention that is offered to aid the visual scan path.

Learner and Richman (1984) state that some individuals, because of ocular motor or binocular instability, tend to skim rather than read in traditional fashion. This is evident in a relatively high grade level performance for individual fixation, regression, and speed components, but may result in poor comprehension due to the technical nature of reading passages. This may also be evident from observing the scan path during reading simulation playback. Some individuals exhibit this pattern because they have a rapid cognitive tempo, and will improve in comprehension by modifying their tempo. Other individuals will find that they have to reduce their reading rate considerably in order to comprehend. When they do try to ramp up their speed without appropriate training, they find themselves having to go back and reread to comprehend. Again, the Visagraph can be used to gain insight into the interactions between cognitive style and visual factors by comparing the graph results to the reading simulation.

Lastly, the Visagraph is a welcome tool for families who home school. One of the principal advantages of home schooling is the ability to individualize and customize a curriculum, an option currently engaging approximately two million children in the United States, according to the National Home Education Research Institute (2012). The Visagraph becomes a valuable addition in documenting the relative rate of progress in the acquisition of ocular-motor-based reading skills. This information is factored together with scores on standardized reading tests. In our center, particularly for parents who are not aware of a child's current reading level, whether or not they are home schooled, we factor together the results of the Woodcock-Johnson Word Identification and Reading Comprehension tests with the Visagraph profile to gain a more complete picture. We work closely with reading specialists who are adept in various methodologies to develop reading performance, and view the Visagraph as essential in documenting visual reading readiness skills.

Case Example

A 12-year-old student in seventh grade, at the time of our first evaluation on December 10, 2009, struggled considerably with reading, and schoolwork was taking considerably longer to complete than it took most of the other classmates. Given the history of the student, we selected a passage for Visagraph recording at Text Level 5, which was two grade levels below the student's current placement. The Visagraph Reading Profile, depicted in Figure 8.1, shows a composite Grade Level Efficiency (GLE) of 1.0 on both recordings, essentially flat lining in all of the composite variables at first grade level.

The student was able to attain a comprehension score of 90 percent. Of particular note is the asymmetry on fixations and regressions:

Fixations/100 words:	L 217	R 229
Regressions/100 words:	L 43	R 52

Assuming that the sensors are properly aligned for the centers of the pupils in both eyes, this extent of difference between the two eyes usually indicates a problem with binocular coordination at near. In this student's case, convergence insufficiency was diagnosed, a type of binocular imbalance that is greater at near than at distance.

We administered a program of optometric vision therapy that resolved the convergence insufficiency, and upon completion on August 12, 2010 (eight months after the pretest was administered), the student's Visagraph Reading Profile was considerably better in all areas as seen in Figure 8.2.

The GLE skyrocketed to 5.9, a 4.9 grade level improvement in an eight-month period of time. Each of the composite eye-movement

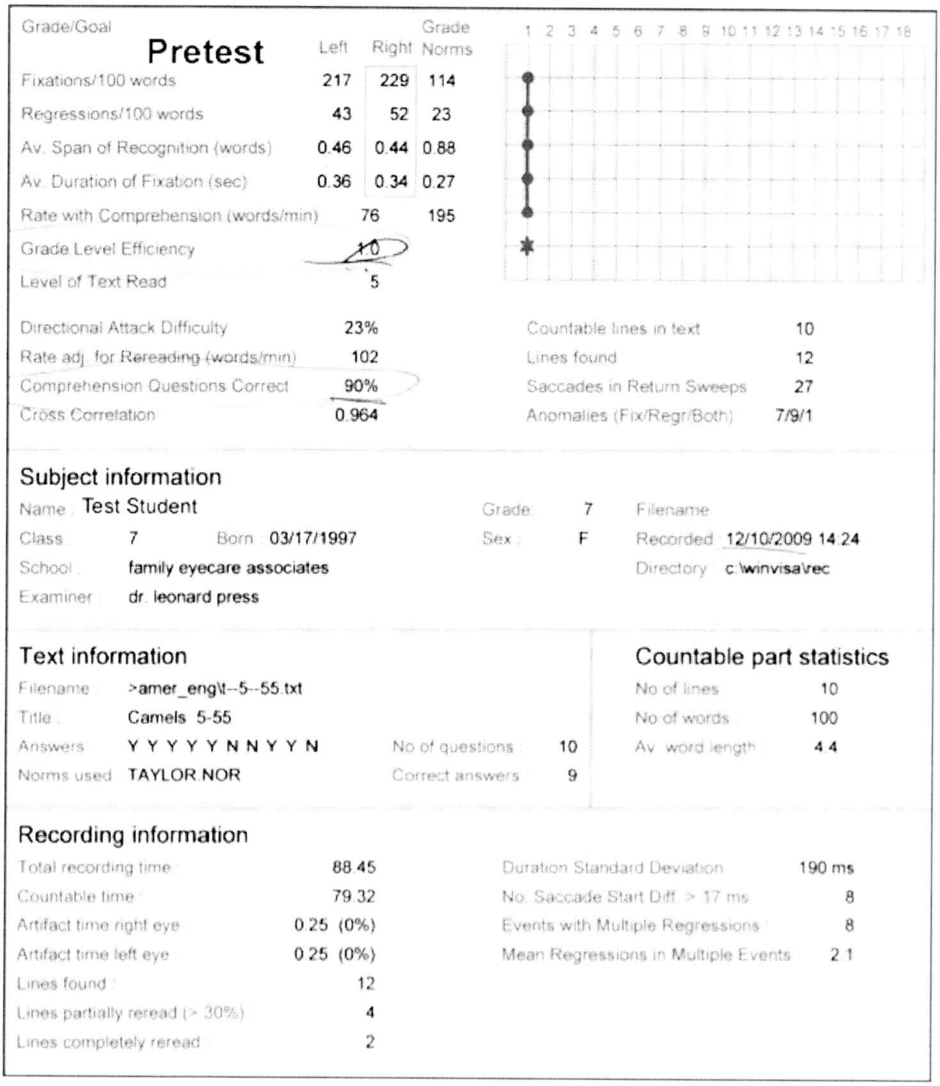

Grade/Goal

Pretest

	Left	Right	Grade Norms
Fixations/100 words	217	229	114
Regressions/100 words	43	52	23
Av. Span of Recognition (words)	0.46	0.44	0.88
Av. Duration of Fixation (sec)	0.36	0.34	0.27
Rate with Comprehension (words/min)	76		195
Grade Level Efficiency	10		
Level of Text Read	5		

Directional Attack Difficulty	23%	Countable lines in text	10
Rate adj. for Rereading (words/min)	102	Lines found	12
Comprehension Questions Correct	90%	Saccades in Return Sweeps	27
Cross Correlation	0.964	Anomalies (Fix/Regr/Both)	7/9/1

Subject information

Name:	Test Student	Grade:	7	Filename	
Class:	7 Born: 03/17/1997	Sex:	F	Recorded:	12/10/2009 14:24
School:	family eyecare associates			Directory:	c:\winvisa\rec
Examiner:	dr. leonard press				

Text information

Filename:	>amer_eng\t--5--55.txt		
Title:	Camels 5-55		
Answers:	Y Y Y Y Y N N Y Y N	No of questions:	10
Norms used:	TAYLOR.NOR	Correct answers:	9

Countable part statistics

No of lines	10
No of words:	100
Av. word length:	4.4

Recording information

Total recording time:	88.45	Duration Standard Deviation	190 ms
Countable time:	79.32	No. Saccade Start Diff. > 17 ms	8
Artifact time right eye:	0.25 (0%)	Events with Multiple Regressions:	8
Artifact time left eye:	0.25 (0%)	Mean Regressions in Multiple Events	2.1
Lines found:	12		
Lines partially reread (> 30%):	4		
Lines completely reread:	2		

Figure 8.1

variables improved significantly. Fixations/100 words were now nearly identical in right and left eyes. Although Regressions/100 words still showed some residual asymmetry, this had little effect on the student's performance. Average Span of Recognition and Average Duration of Fixation were identical in both eyes. Directional Attack Difficulty improved from 23 percent to 15 percent and the Rate adjusted for Reading (words/min) improved from 102 to 186.

Grade/Goal **Posttest**

	Left	Right	Grade Norms
Fixations/100 words	129	128	109
Regressions/100 words	19	12	21
Av. Span of Recognition (words)	0.78	0.78	0.92
Av. Duration of Fixation (sec)	0.25	0.25	0.27
Rate with Comprehension (words/min)	186		204
Grade Level Efficiency	5.9		
Level of Text Read	5		

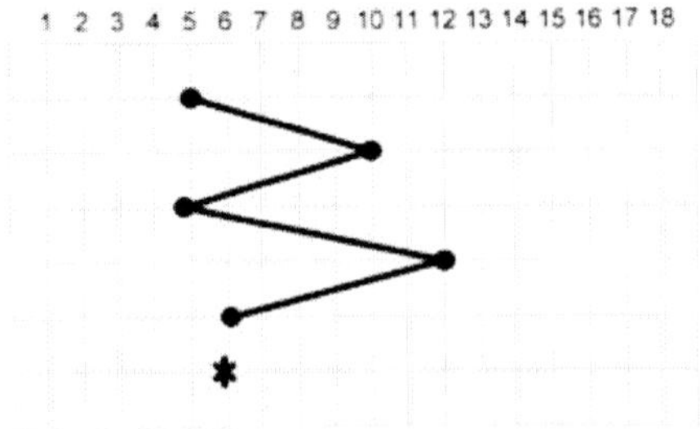

Directional Attack Difficulty	15%	Countable lines in text	10
Rate adj. for Rereading (words/min)	186	Lines found	8
Comprehension Questions Correct	80%	Saccades in Return Sweeps	11
Cross Correlation	0.835	Anomalies (Fix/Regr/Both)	0/1/12

Subject information

Name :	Test Student	Grade :	8	Filename :	
Class :	8 Born : 03/17/1997	Sex :	F	Recorded :	08/12/2010 18:10
School :	family eyecare associates			Directory :	c:\winvisa\rec
Examiner :	dr. leonard press				

Text information

Filename :	>amer_eng\t--5--54.txt			No of lines :	10
Title :	Whales 5-54			No of words :	100
Answers :	N N Y Y Y N Y Y N Y	No of questions :	10	Av. word length :	4.2
Norms used :	TAYLOR.NOR	Correct answers :	8		

Countable part statistics

Recording information

Total recording time :	40.20	Duration Standard Deviation :	139 ms
Countable time :	32.32	No. Saccade Start Diff. > 17 ms:	10
Artifact time right eye :	4.77 (15%)	Events with Multiple Regressions :	0
Artifact time left eye :	4.77 (15%)	Mean Regressions in Multiple Events :	
Lines found :	8		
Lines partially reread (> 30%) :	0		
Lines completely reread :	0		

Figure 8.2

The student's father was delighted with his child's improvement. As other reading interventions had been tried before with little success, and no other interventions were undertaken during this time period, we were confident that the Visagraph results objectively supported the transfer of optometric vision therapy to the student's ocular motor efficiency in reading.

Doug Major, O.D., FCOVD
El Paso de Robles School
Paso Robles, CA
805–238–1001
Los Osos, CA
805–528–5333
Vision Therapy Program

In September, 1988, the office of Criminal Planning approved funds for a pilot study at the El Paso de Robles School to demonstrate the need for and effects of vision therapy on the student wards. In the subsequent two years, the program was unanimously approved for further funding, and ESEA funds were made available after the three-year maximum was completed. Studies in Plainfield, Indiana; Denver, Colorado; San Bernardino Juvenile Hall in California; and others have shown the positive effect of vision therapy intervention.

Critics have questioned the previous research results citing poor experimental design and/or insufficient sample size. Our study at the PRYA was designed and monitored by the Statistical Department of the California Youth Authority. The program was also audited by the OCJP.

We designed a controlled research program to test the effects of treatment in the areas of:

Literacy: The standard subjective measure of reading ability for an institutional population is the TABE. Because of the variability of response of the wards we also chose an objective measure of reading efficiency, the Visagraph. This testing instrument records eye movement using infrared sensors as the student looks across the text. Good reading ability is essential for success at the school and upon parole.

Behavior Modification: Behavior reports were compiled on each ward of the PRYA. They are totaled according to severity. Level A is less serious and Level B is more serious. Fewer behavior problems reduce management costs and allow more productive activities while being detained.

Recidivism: The State of California OBITS system tracks youth involvement with the judicial system in days. Reduced recidivism is the ultimate goal of all PRYA activities.

Self Esteem: Wards complete the Tennessee Self-Concept Scale before treatment and upon leaving the institution. Good self-concept has been shown to be a vital factor for parole success.

Basic Overview of the Vision Therapy Program

Background

- 2,016 wards received a vision-screening test. Of these, 560 were chosen to participate in a vision-training program; 276 wards completed vision therapy and the rest are in the control group.
- Six ward aides were trained and have assisted with the program, totaling 5,000+ service hours.
- Technical assistance was provided by Sharon Winter, Ph.D., Research Division, Department of the California Youth Authority.

Findings Update 1/92

Literacy: 188 of the 276 experimental group wards (68 percent) increased their reading literacy by 2.0 grade levels or higher within a two-month period. Of the 284 control group wards, 102 (36 percent) were able to do the same.

Table 8.1

Average Grade Level Change (over a two-month period)			
Group	TABE Score	Visagraph® Reading Rate	Visagraph® Visual Efficiency
Experimental (276 wards)	+1.2	+2.4 grades	+2.6 grades
Control (201 wards)	+0.6	+0.12 grades	-0.01 grades

Behavior Reports were collected two months prior to the wards beginning therapy and then were collected two months after the wards had completed their therapy.

The experimental group wards had 74 fewer total behavior reports (8 percent decrease), while the control group wards had 226 more total behavior reports (33 percent increase).

The experimental group wards had 14 fewer Level B behavior reports (47 percent decrease), while the control group wards had four fewer reports (17 percent decrease).

Recidivism: 108 wards from the experimental group were paroled and 50 had 99 percent to 100 percent "good street time" as tracked by OBITS (46 percent). Ninety-five wards from the control group were paroled and 33 had 99 percent to 100 percent "good street time" (34 percent).

All incoming wards are now screened for potential visually-related learning problems along with regular academic testing and the TABE. We have found that over 90 percent of the students reading at seventh grade level or below have a visual deficit in one or more of the following areas:

Refractive Error: These are problems such as near or farsightedness and astigmatism that could be corrected by glasses. As others have found, most of the wards who need correction are farsighted with or without astigmatism. Often these individuals can pass a distance 20/20 chart but have great difficulty focusing up close.

Binocular or Eye Teaming Problems: If the eyes don't work together properly, double vision and/or eyestrain can result. We have found a number of our wards cannot converge or cross their eyes well. This adversely affects any prolonged near work.

Accommodation or Focusing Dysfunction: To be efficient, the eye must be able to have clear focus at all distances, quickly and freely. We have found a number of wards have difficulty with sustained focus at the reading distance.

Eye Tracking or Scanning: Nothing reveals more about a person's ability to process visual information than a careful eye-movement evaluation. With the Visagraph Eye Movement Recording system, we assess the number of times the eye stops per word, the direction of the eyes' movements, number of lines skipped or reread, and the speed of the eyes while reading.

One of the incoming wards was asked if he had trouble reading. "Yes," admitted the new resident of the California Youth Authority's El Paso de Robles School.

"Well, you can't focus," a vision therapist told him during the screening tests offered to all new wards. "You can't see the letters."

The youngster looked surprised at this. "You mean I'm not stupid?" That's a common reaction among the school's residents who participate in an experimental vision therapy program developed by Dr. Douglas L. Major, a Paso Robles optometrist.

"Some people might think they can't read because they're dumb," said Solomon Adegbenro, a CYA ward and graduate of the program. "It could be because their eyes hurt or they can't see. This program helps you use your eyes better."

Barry Tannen, OD, FCOVD, FAAO
EyeCare Professionals, PC
Hamilton Square, New Jersey
609–581–5755
btannenod@aol.com

Clinical Use of the Visagraph in an Optometric Clinic

In our practice, we specialize in visually-related learning problems. Therefore, we are frequently called upon to evaluate whether dysfunctions of the visual system are causally related to learning problems. Frequently, we are requested to assess individuals with reported reading difficulties. Accompanying symptoms can include: loss of place when reading, skipping of words, headaches, and moderately or severely reduced reading speed. We rely primarily on the Visagraph Eye Movement Recording System. This is a commercially available testing system that objectively records reading eye movement with computer automation. It compares the results to a large standardized population over a range of established parameters. Hence, it directly measures and assesses eye movements during actual reading, and also measures comprehension level.

From an optometric standpoint, we tend to attribute reading problems to two primary factors: oculomotor and language. Patients with oculomotor dysfunction tend to perform on or close to grade level on standardized reading tests. However, their symptoms suggest an oculomotor inefficiency. These symptoms include loss of place and skipping of words when reading, a reduced reading rate, as well as a difference in the performance of the two eyes.

In order to determine whether the reading problem is primarily language based or oculomotor based, we have changed the standard protocol. In addition to testing patients at their independent reading level, we also test them at a significantly reduced text level (up to five grade levels below when possible). We have found that patients who perform poorly when measured at their independent reading level and at the reduced text level are the patients whose reading difficulties are significantly due to problems with their oculomotor system, and who respond most positively to optometric vision therapy. Usually after vision therapy we find that these patients have significant improvement in symptoms, school performance, and Visagraph results. The following Visagraph Reading profiles are indicative of the types of results we often achieve pre- and post-vision therapy.

Pre-Vision Therapy Fifth Grade

In Figure 8.3 of a student report, the Cross Correlation below 90 percent suggests visual/functional problems. Also a Directional Attack Difficulty above 15 percent and the difference in the number of Fixations and Regressions likewise suggests visual/functional problems.

Post-Vision Therapy Sixth Grade

Eight months later, after completing training, the same student's Visagraph posttest report, shown in Figure 8.4, indicates an improved Cross Correlation above 90 percent, suggesting satisfactory visual/functional proficiency despite a slightly higher-than-desired Directional Attack Difficulty. Further, the number of Fixations and Regressions, Duration of Fixation, and Reading Rate indicate the student has made substantial progress in reading achievement.

Charles E. Shearer, OD
Bernell Corporation
Mishawaka, Indiana
574-259-2070
www.bernell.com
bernellconsult@aol.com

I have been using the Visagraph for over 12 years. It is one of the most valuable instruments in my optometric practice and it is an invaluable tool in evaluating visually-related reading problems. I first purchased the instrument as a means of objectively determining if a

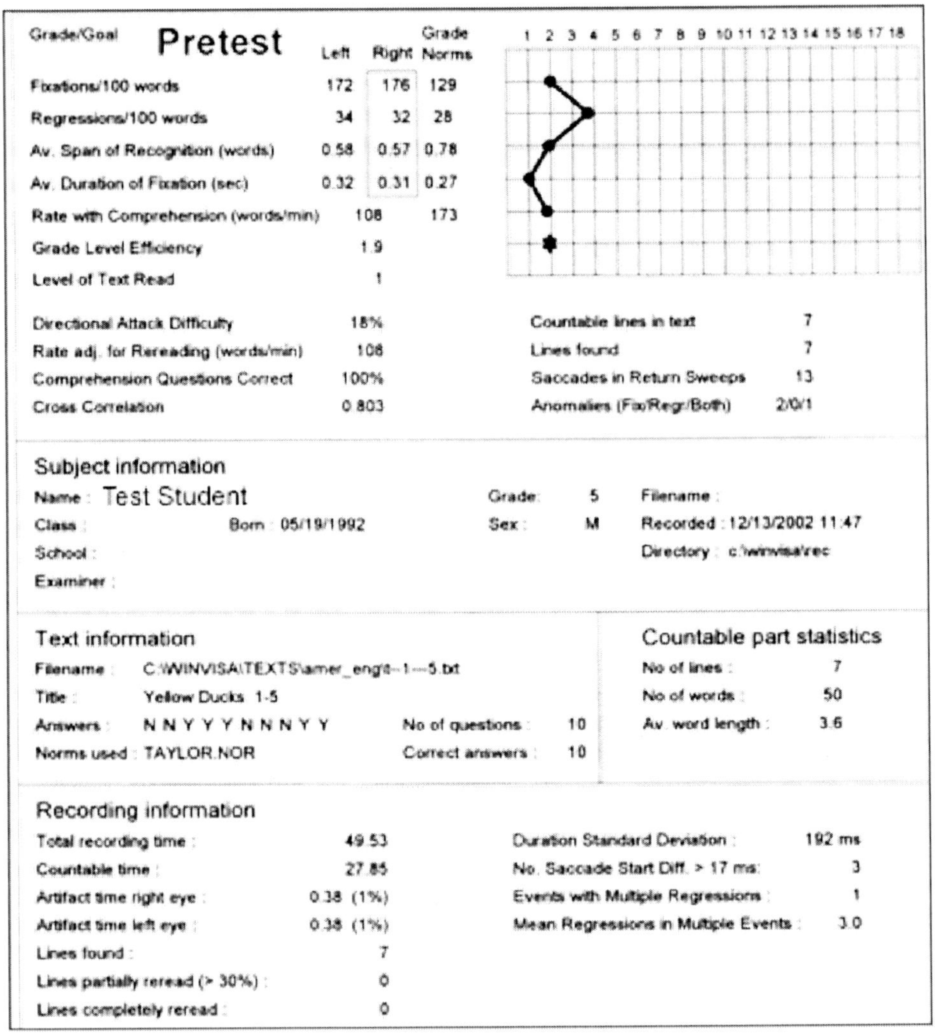

Grade/Goal **Pretest**	Left	Right	Grade Norms
Fixations/100 words	172	176	129
Regressions/100 words	34	32	28
Av. Span of Recognition (words)	0.58	0.57	0.78
Av. Duration of Fixation (sec)	0.32	0.31	0.27
Rate with Comprehension (words/min)	108		173
Grade Level Efficiency	1.9		
Level of Text Read	1		

Directional Attack Difficulty	18%	Countable lines in text	7
Rate adj. for Rereading (words/min)	108	Lines found	7
Comprehension Questions Correct	100%	Saccades in Return Sweeps	13
Cross Correlation	0.803	Anomalies (Fix/Regr/Both)	2/0/1

Subject information

Name : Test Student Grade: 5 Filename :
Class : Born : 05/19/1992 Sex : M Recorded : 12/13/2002 11:47
School : Directory : c:\winvisa\rec
Examiner :

Text information

Filename : C:\WINVISA\TEXTS\amer_eng\t--1---5.txt
Title : Yellow Ducks 1-5
Answers : N N Y Y Y N N N Y Y No of questions : 10
Norms used : TAYLOR.NOR Correct answers : 10

Countable part statistics

No of lines : 7
No of words : 50
Av. word length : 3.6

Recording information

Total recording time :	49.53	Duration Standard Deviation :	192 ms
Countable time :	27.85	No. Saccade Start Diff. > 17 ms:	3
Artifact time right eye :	0.38 (1%)	Events with Multiple Regressions :	1
Artifact time left eye :	0.38 (1%)	Mean Regressions in Multiple Events :	3.0
Lines found :	7		
Lines partially reread (> 30%) :	0		
Lines completely reread :	0		

Figure 8.3

colored filter would affect a child's reading performance. I would test each child with a reading problem with and without a blue filter. If a significant difference in reading speed occurred, I would tint their lenses. This objective test was extremely essential in demonstrating the effect to parents and children alike.

I next used it to decide if low-plus reading glasses would improve reading ability. I made up a pair of +.50, +.75 and +1.00 reading lens-

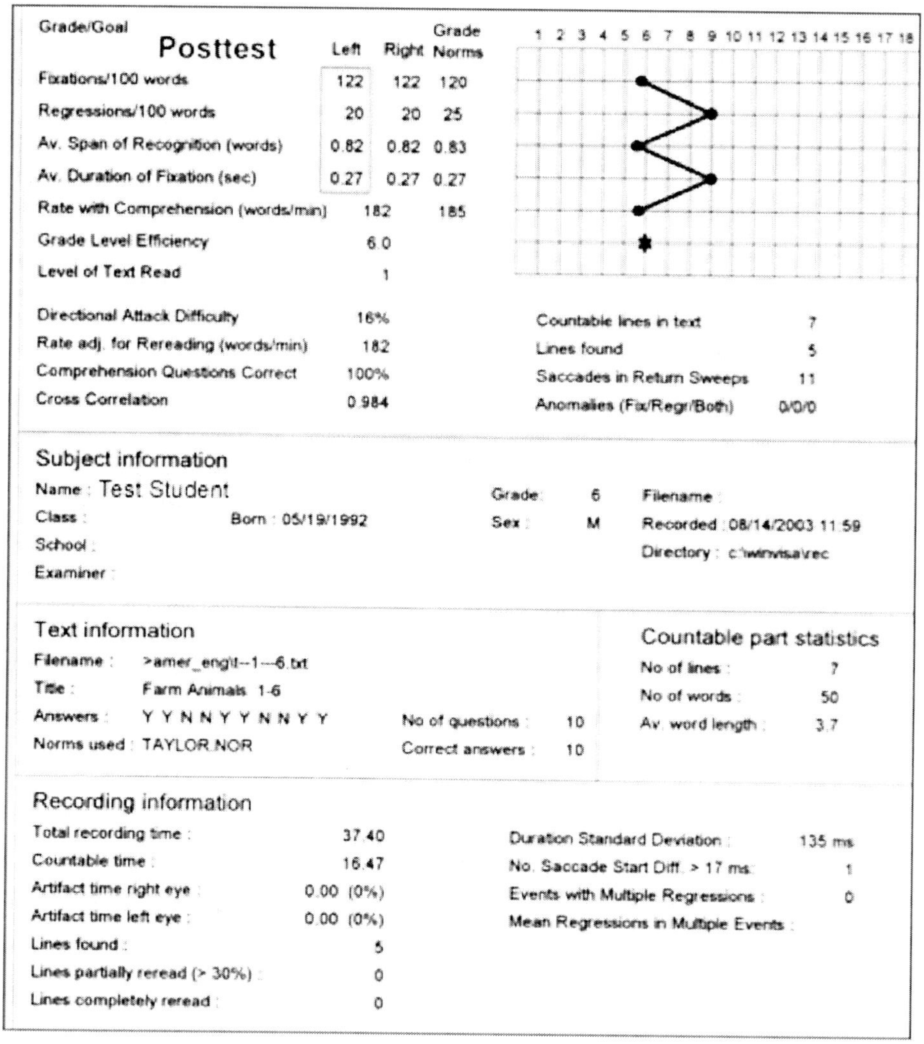
Grade/Goal
Posttest

	Left	Right	Grade Norms
Fixations/100 words	122	122	120
Regressions/100 words	20	20	25
Av. Span of Recognition (words)	0.82	0.82	0.83
Av. Duration of Fixation (sec)	0.27	0.27	0.27
Rate with Comprehension (words/min)	182		185
Grade Level Efficiency	6.0		
Level of Text Read	1		

Directional Attack Difficulty 16%
Rate adj. for Rereading (words/min) 182
Comprehension Questions Correct 100%
Cross Correlation 0.984

Countable lines in text 7
Lines found 5
Saccades in Return Sweeps 11
Anomalies (Fix/Regr/Both) 0/0/0

Subject information
Name: Test Student
Class:
Born: 05/19/1992
School:
Examiner:
Grade: 6
Sex: M
Filename:
Recorded: 08/14/2003 11:59
Directory: c:\winvisa\rec

Text information
Filename: >amer_eng\t--1--6.txt
Title: Farm Animals 1-6
Answers: Y Y N N Y Y N N Y Y
Norms used: TAYLOR.NOR
No of questions: 10
Correct answers: 10

Countable part statistics
No of lines: 7
No of words: 50
Av. word length: 3.7

Recording information
Total recording time: 37.40
Countable time: 16.47
Artifact time right eye: 0.00 (0%)
Artifact time left eye: 0.00 (0%)
Lines found: 5
Lines partially reread (> 30%): 0
Lines completely reread: 0
Duration Standard Deviation: 135 ms
No. Saccade Start Diff. > 17 ms: 1
Events with Multiple Regressions: 0
Mean Regressions in Multiple Events:

Figure 8.4

es with anti-reflective lenses and tested with and without the plus lenses to see if there was a significant change in performance to warrant prescribing lenses. Parents particularly liked this as they could immediately see the benefit of purchasing reading glasses for their children.

I will run a Visagraph on any child who has a complaint of loss of place, skipping rows, rereading rows, or word reversals. Word reversals may be either perceptual or mechanical in nature. If a child skips over the word "was," then realizes that he or she did that and goes back to see it, he or she is now moving from right to left instead of left to right. This may cause him or her to see the "s" first and read the word as "saw." This is less common with individual letter reversals such as "b" and "d."

Another common complaint of a saccadic eye movement problem is skipping over words and substituting a word in their place. This is particularly true of little words as they are easily overshot. These readers will often simply replace the skipped over word with one that just makes sense, such as "from" instead of "for."

The Visagraph is also a great practice management tool. I always invite the parent to quietly observe the testing. They are not allowed to comment or help in any way during the test, although some will try. If we sense that the parent is making the child nervous or is in any way affecting the test, we repeat the test with them out of the room. This is rarely a problem, though, and it is worthwhile for the parent to see what is going on and why. Once the test is completed, we discuss the results right away. The most useful tools for this are the summary report and the Simulation. The Simulation roughly illustrates with a moving curser how the child moved his or her eyes while reading the words. This can often be very dramatic in nature to the point where it has brought tears to the eyes of many a parent. We often hear the comment, "No wonder he is having a reading problem."

I personally put a large emphasis on the duration of fixation score, or as I explain it to the parent: how quickly the child understands what he sees. Visual processing speed and accuracy is a trainable skill. Tachistoscoptic training, for example, can greatly improve it. How quickly and accurately the child sees is indirectly related to reading performance.

The other aspect of the Viasgraph, as a practice builder, is the number of school referrals we receive after doing an in-service program and/or demonstrating at the local school. I often give schools a DEM test and teach them how to screen for eye-movement problems. A well-placed letter or report back to the teacher or reading specialist never hurts, either. Teachers often see reading problems that they cannot explain. We can provide a logical and objective reason for what they are seeing the child do. Many times this leads to one of those "ah ha!" moments, like a light bulb going off in the teacher's head.

There are many aspects and complicated processes that go into the visual part of reading: focus, eye alignment, visual acuity, and visual processing speed, to list a few. But I do not feel any are more important than accurate and precise eye movements. The Visagraph is a tool that lets a doctor diagnosis the problem, direct the therapy, and measure the improvement.

The Visagraph pretest and posttest results, shown in the following images, demonstrate the improvements that can be achieved.

In Figure 8.5, a grade three student's pretest indicates:

- FRP skills are much lower than grade three norms
- Reading Rate is 61 words per minute
- Grade Level Efficiency is only 1.0.

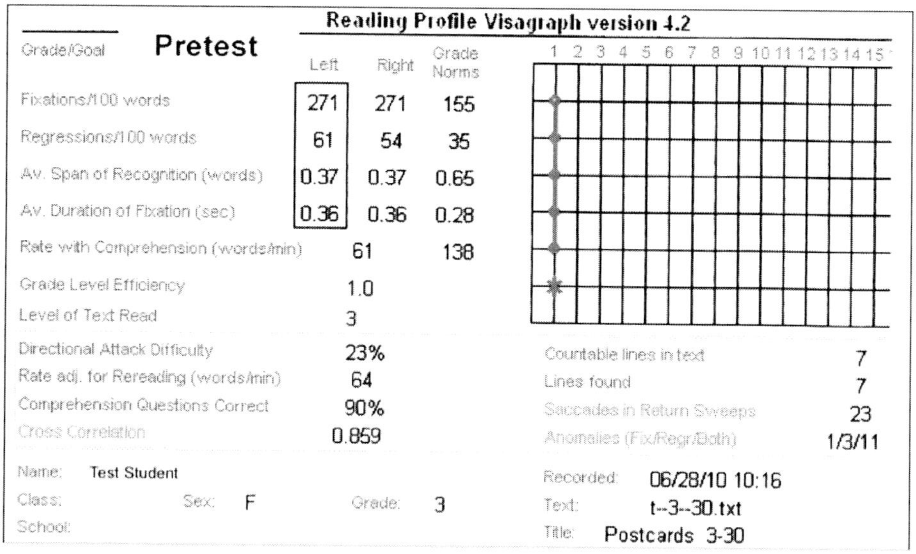

Reading Profile Visagraph version 4.2

Grade/Goal: Pretest	Left	Right	Grade Norms
Fixations/100 words	271	271	155
Regressions/100 words	61	54	35
Av. Span of Recognition (words)	0.37	0.37	0.65
Av. Duration of Fixation (sec)	0.36	0.36	0.28
Rate with Comprehension (words/min)	61		138
Grade Level Efficiency	1.0		
Level of Text Read	3		
Directional Attack Difficulty	23%		
Rate adj. for Rereading (words/min)	64		
Comprehension Questions Correct	90%		
Cross Correlation	0.859		

Countable lines in text	7
Lines found	7
Saccades in Return Sweeps	23
Anomalies (Fix/Regr/Both)	1/3/11

Name: Test Student
Class: Sex: F Grade: 3
School:
Recorded: 06/28/10 10:16
Text: t--3--30.txt
Title: Postcards 3-30

Figure 8.5

In Figure 8.6, the same student (now in grade four) achieved the following posttest results:

- FRP skills are better than grade four level norms
- Reading Rate is now 144 words per minute
- Grade Level Efficiency is now 3.5, which is an improvement at two-and-a-half grade levels higher than the pretest administered a year earlier.

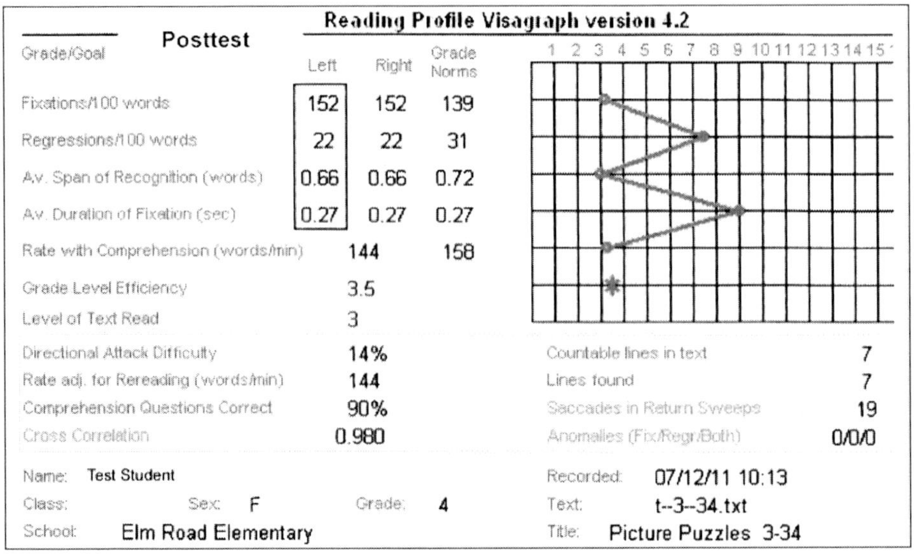

Reading Profile Visagraph version 4.2

Grade/Goal **Posttest**

	Left	Right	Grade Norms
Fixations/100 words	152	152	139
Regressions/100 words	22	22	31
Av. Span of Recognition (words)	0.66	0.66	0.72
Av. Duration of Fixation (sec)	0.27	0.27	0.27
Rate with Comprehension (words/min)	144		158
Grade Level Efficiency	3.5		
Level of Text Read	3		

Directional Attack Difficulty	14%
Rate adj. for Rereading (words/min)	144
Comprehension Questions Correct	90%
Cross Correlation	0.980
Countable lines in text	7
Lines found	7
Saccades in Return Sweeps	19
Anomalies (Fix/Regr/Both)	0/0/0

Name: Test Student
Class: Sex: F Grade: 4
School: Elm Road Elementary
Recorded: 07/12/11 10:13
Text: t--3--34.txt
Title: Picture Puzzles 3-34

Figure 8.6

In Figure 8.7, a grade three student's pretest indicates:

- FRP skills are well lower than grade three norms
- Reading Rate is marked at 91 words per minute
- Grade Level Efficiency is 1.1.

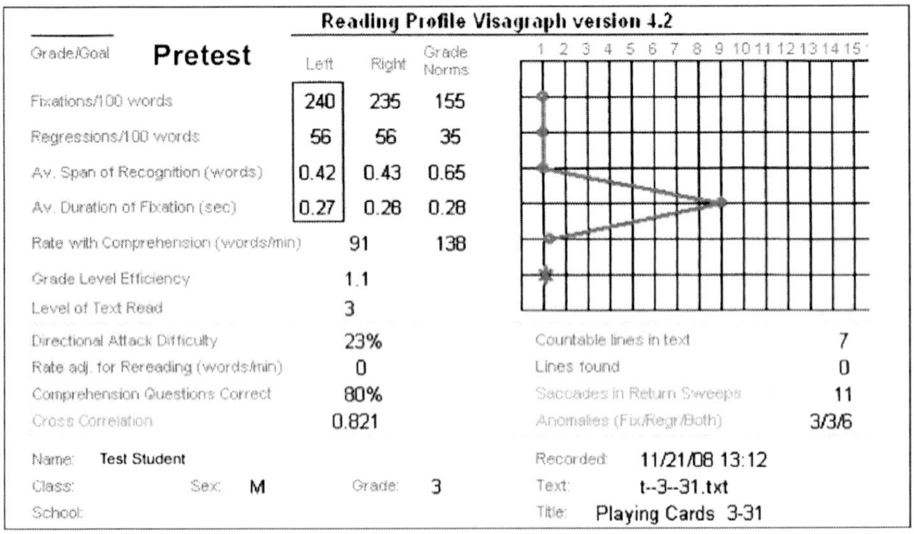

Reading Profile Visagraph version 4.2

Grade/Goal **Pretest**

	Left	Right	Grade Norms
Fixations/100 words	240	235	155
Regressions/100 words	56	56	35
Av. Span of Recognition (words)	0.42	0.43	0.65
Av. Duration of Fixation (sec)	0.27	0.28	0.28
Rate with Comprehension (words/min)	91		138
Grade Level Efficiency	1.1		
Level of Text Read	3		

Directional Attack Difficulty	23%
Rate adj. for Rereading (words/min)	0
Comprehension Questions Correct	80%
Cross Correlation	0.821
Countable lines in text	7
Lines found	0
Saccades in Return Sweeps	11
Anomalies (Fix/Regr/Both)	3/3/6

Name: Test Student
Class: Sex: M Grade: 3
School:
Recorded: 11/21/08 13:12
Text: t--3--31.txt
Title: Playing Cards 3-31

Figure 8.7

In Figure 8.8, the same student (now in grade four) achieved the following posttest results:

- FRP skills are better than grade four level norms
- Reading Rate is now 192 words per minute without rereading
- Grade Level Efficiency is now 7.5.

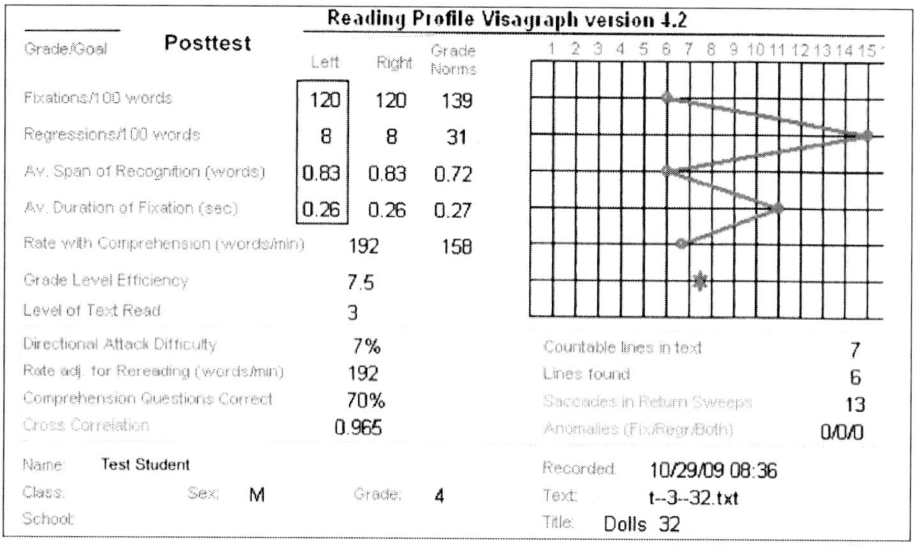

Figure 8.8

In Figure 8.9, a grade five student's pretest indicates:

- FRP skills are lower than grade five norms
- Reading Rate is 124 words per minute
- Grade Level Efficiency is only 3.0.

In Figure 8.10, the same student (now in grade six) achieved the following posttest results:

- FRP skills are better than grade six level norms
- Reading Rate is now 162 words per minute
- Grade Level Efficiency is now 5.5.

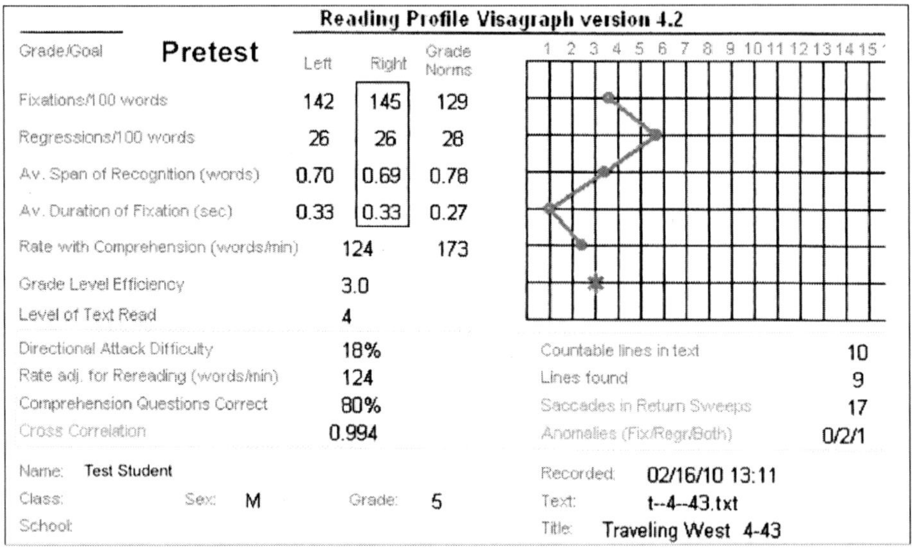

Figure 8.9

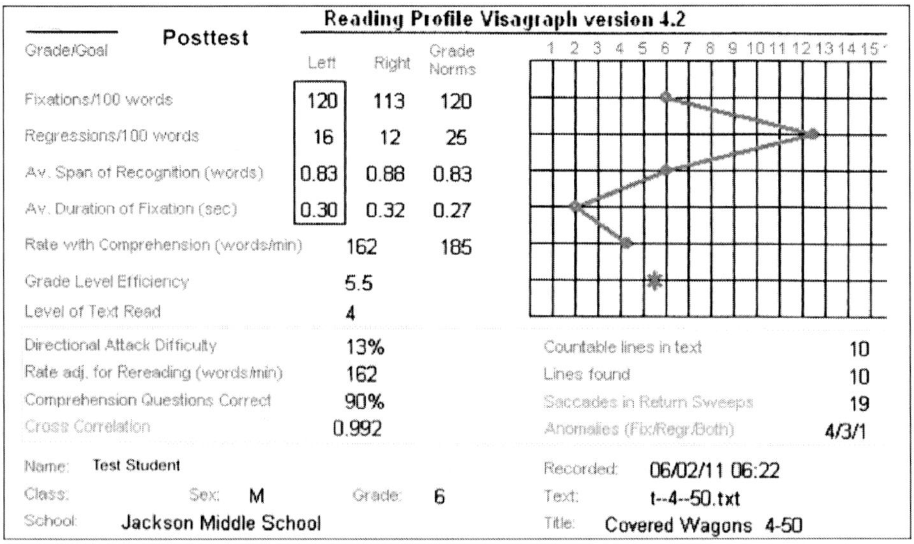

Figure 8.10

In Figure 8.11, a grade seven student's pretest indicates:

- FRP skills are lower than grade seven norms
- Reading Rate is 115 words per minute
- Grade Level Efficiency is only 2.4.

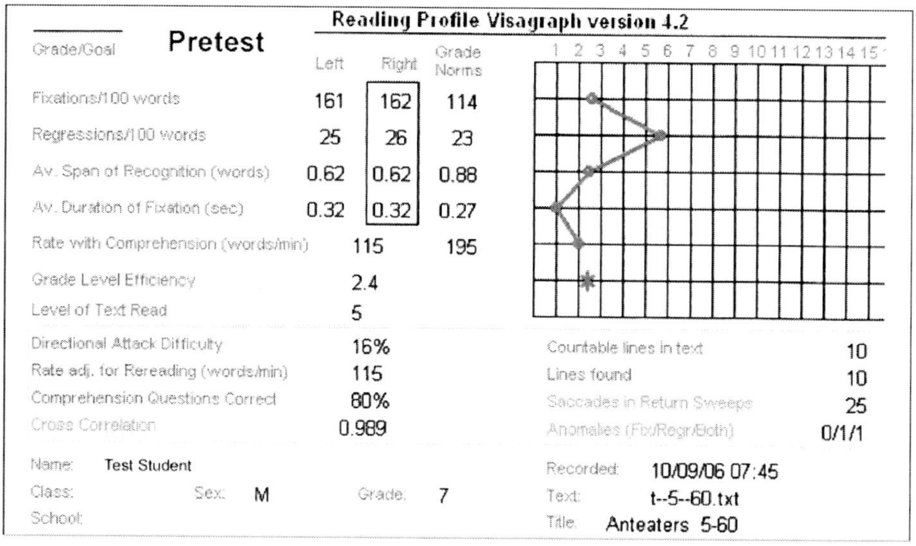

Figure 8.11

In Figure 8.12, the same student (now in grade eight) achieved the following posttest results:

- FRP skills are at grade eight level norms
- Reading Rate is now 194 words per minute
- Grade Level Efficiency is now 7.2.

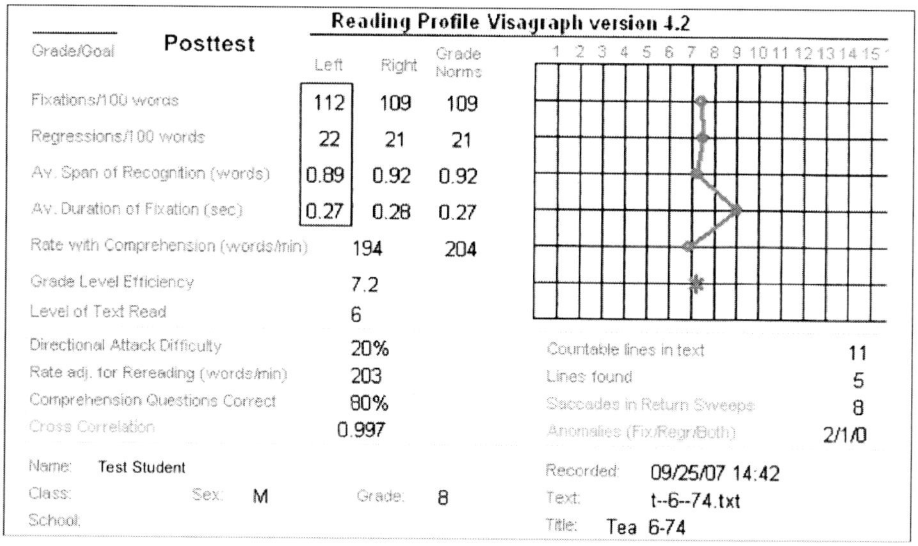

Figure 8.12

Darrell G. Schlange, OD, DOS, FAAO
Associate Professor of Optometry, Pediatrics/Binocular Vision
Illinois College of Optometry (http://www.ico.edu)
Illinois Eye Institute (http://iei.ico.edu)
Chicago, Illinois
Office: 312–949–7284
Cell: 708–254–7446
dschlang@ico.edu

Uses of the Visagraph at the Illinois College of Optometry and Illinois Eye Institute

The Illinois College of Optometry and Illinois Eye Institute (IEI) have an extensive eye-movement clinic that is used in didactics, clinical patient care, and research. The emphasis is to provide clinical experiences for our students and also develop a patient-centered and evidence-based clinic and research program.

The didactic curriculum provides all students with hands-on experience, administering the Visagraph on fellow students and having the procedure completed on themselves. We have six Visagraph units for laboratory experiments during the second-year ocular motility course. The clinicians develop experience with the clinical procedures and interpretation during their third- or fourth-year rotation in the pediatrics/binocular vision service. Seminars are presented for our pediatric residents and senior students, emphasizing binocular vision and ocular motility cases, evidence-based research, and clinical skills and knowledge.

Our clinical program includes an Eye-Movement Clinic (EMC) for patients referred from other IEI services and also from outside medical and educational facilities. Visagraph procedures are provided when reported signs and symptoms including:

- Visually-related reading problems
- Binocular vision problems during reading
- Symptoms of excessive head movements and losing place while reading.
- Poor reading fluency and oculomotor dysfunction (OMD)
- Problems with visual development, visual perception, and visual attention

- Pre-therapy and post-therapy to monitor VT progress
- Special needs: autism, nystagmus, strabismus, traumatic brain injury, etc.

Other routine saccadic and fixation tests provided in this clinic include the King-Devick Test, Developmental Eye Movement Test, and the Maples NSUCO Test. These results may be integrated with a Visual Efficiency Exam, a Visual Information Processing Exam, and Visual Attention Tests. The FixTest and FixTrain procedures by Fischer use a gap and overlap test paradigm for assessing fixations, prosaccades, and anti-saccades.

The Visagraph Reading and Numbers tests provide a dynamic assessment of near vision function during active reading and sequential visual processing of numbers, letters, and words. The Numbers Test is also used for non-verbal patients or those unable to read at grade one level. The Visual Skills Test is used to evaluate fixations and saccadic control, accuracy, and speed, commonly in the preschool, kindergarten, or first-grade child. We usually combine a Visagraph Reading Test with the Numbers Test to evaluate reading eye movements with and without words and text. We generally follow our Visagraph Protocol for most patients.

We have a myriad of active research studies investigating, among others, eye movements with visual attention; anti-saccades; traumatic brain injury; neuro-ocular disease; pre/post-treatment (vision therapy or glasses); and sports-related eye movements for professional, college, and high school soccer and basketball teams. Nystagmus and pupil studies use the ISCAN, a remote and/or head-mounted camera simultaneously recording horizontal and vertical movements at a sampling frequency up to 240 Hz, linear range +/- 20 deg., and spatial resolution of 0.3 deg.

The visual function test gives insight into binocularity, with tests for cross-correlation, saccadic start differences, anomalies, saccades on new line refixations, standard deviation, and comparison between right and left eyes. Saccadic accuracy is considered with grade-appropriate fixations, regressions, standard deviation, saccadic ratio, and rate. The Grade Level Equivalent gives a good global index that patients, parents, and teachers easily understand. Reading fluency is a blend of both reading ability and visual/functional coordination.

The information provided by this battery of tests includes: a print-out of the graph recordings and a reading profile of the results; a read-

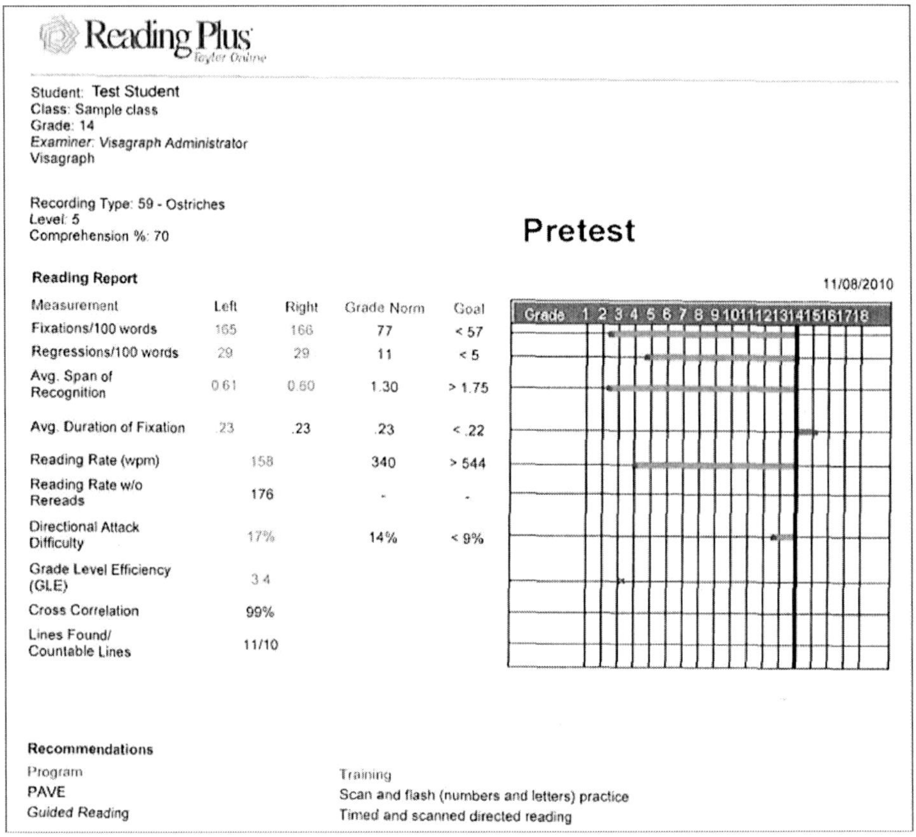

Reading Plus Taylor Online

Student: Test Student
Class: Sample class
Grade: 14
Examiner: Visagraph Administrator
Visagraph

Recording Type: 59 - Ostriches
Level: 5
Comprehension %: 70

Pretest

Reading Report

11/08/2010

Measurement	Left	Right	Grade Norm	Goal
Fixations/100 words	165	166	77	< 57
Regressions/100 words	29	29	11	< 5
Avg. Span of Recognition	0.61	0.60	1.30	> 1.75
Avg. Duration of Fixation	.23	.23	.23	< .22
Reading Rate (wpm)	158		340	> 544
Reading Rate w/o Rereads	176		-	-
Directional Attack Difficulty	17%		14%	< 9%
Grade Level Efficiency (GLE)	3.4			
Cross Correlation	99%			
Lines Found/ Countable Lines	11/10			

Recommendations

Program	Training
PAVE	Scan and flash (numbers and letters) practice
Guided Reading	Timed and scanned directed reading

Figure 8.13

ing eye movements Grade Level Efficiency score; a Developmental Level of Saccades, Fixations, and Reading fluency; the Span of Recognition and Fixation Duration to Process Visual Information; and Binocular Vision Anomalies occurring during dynamic reading.

A detailed report of the results is provided and discussed with the patient, parent, and referring individual. A list of recommendations and treatment options are given. Treatment may include a combination of corrective lenses, vision therapy, adaptive techniques, and recommendations for the school and classroom. We have a report form that has findings and interpretation for all results. We will commonly have a teleconference with interested parties in the case. A copy is also provided to teachers, therapists, and referring doctors.

Figure 8.13 of a pre-therapy recording is from an adult patient with traumatic brain injury (TBI) receiving treatment following a head con-

Reading Plus

Student: Test Student
Class: Sample class
Grade: 13
Examiner: Visagraph Administrator
Visagraph

Recording Type: 59 - Ostriches
Level: 5
Comprehension %: 80

Intermediary Test

Reading Report

05/09/2011

Measurement	Left	Right	Grade Norm	Goal
Fixations/100 words	132	132	90	< 57
Regressions/100 words	14	12	15	< 5
Avg. Span of Recognition	0.76	0.76	1.11	> 1.75
Avg. Duration of Fixation	.21	.21	.24	< .22
Reading Rate (wpm)	214		280	> 448
Reading Rate w/o Rereads	231		-	-
Directional Attack Difficulty	11%		17%	< 9%
Grade Level Efficiency (GLE)	7.3			
Cross Correlation	98%			
Lines Found/ Countable Lines	11/10			

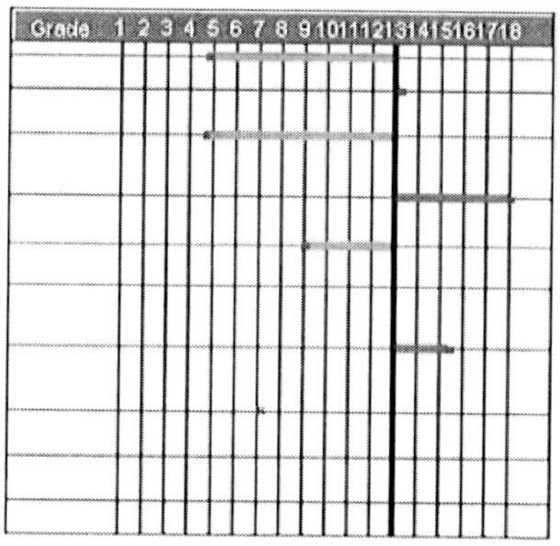

Recommendations

Program	Training
PAVE	Scan and flash (numbers and letters) practice
Guided Reading	Timed and scanned directed reading

Figure 8.14

cussion. Key findings include: excessive fixations and regressions; poor directional attack and saccadic accuracy; reduced recognition span; long fixation duration; poor age-level rate and GLE.

After 20 weekly sessions during six months of vision therapy, another Visagraph recording was done on the same adult patient. In the intermediary test, as seen Figure 8.14, improvement was significant and many FRP skills, such as pronounced reductions in fixations and regressions, were achieved. The patient was compliant with the computer-based therapy program that included both weekly office sessions and daily home activities.

Figure 8.15 shows the recording that was taken after an additional 18 sessions at the completion of one-and-a-half years of therapy. The patient achieved overall improvement in all areas treated including: decreased fixations, regressions, and directional attack; increased span

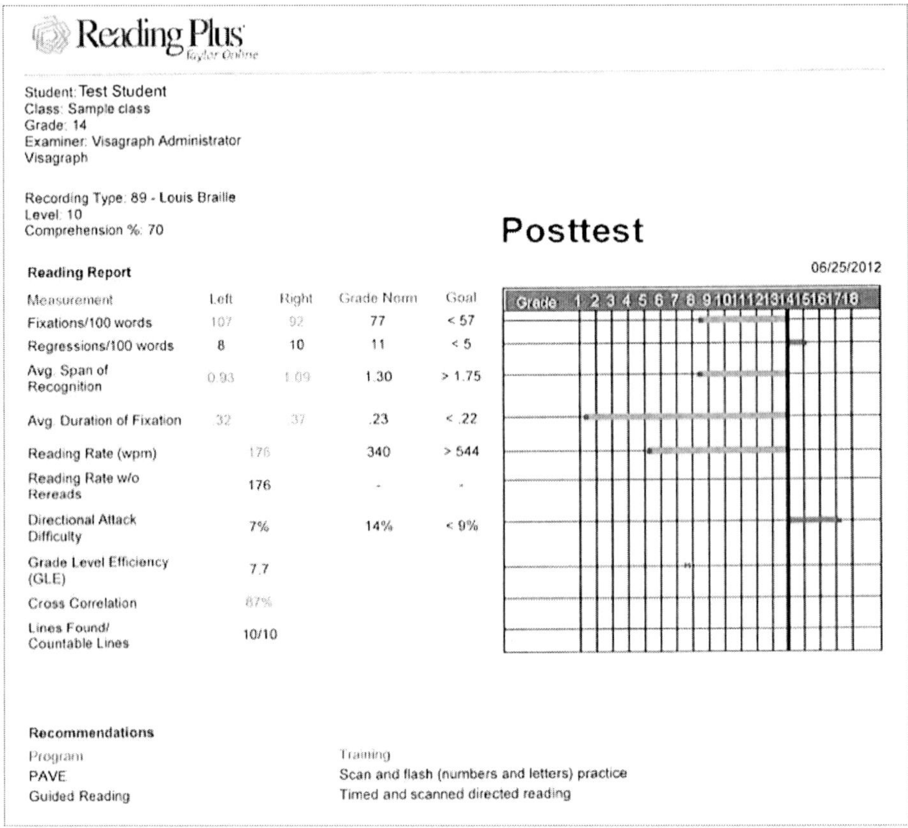

Reading Plus
Taylor Online

Student: Test Student
Class: Sample class
Grade: 14
Examiner: Visagraph Administrator
Visagraph

Recording Type: 89 - Louis Braille
Level: 10
Comprehension %: 70

Posttest

06/25/2012

Reading Report

Measurement	Left	Right	Grade Norm	Goal
Fixations/100 words	107	92	77	< 57
Regressions/100 words	8	10	11	< 5
Avg. Span of Recognition	0.93	1.09	1.30	> 1.75
Avg. Duration of Fixation	.32	.37	.23	< .22
Reading Rate (wpm)	176		340	> 544
Reading Rate w/o Rereads	176		-	-
Directional Attack Difficulty	7%		14%	< 9%
Grade Level Efficiency (GLE)	7.7			
Cross Correlation	87%			
Lines Found/ Countable Lines	10/10			

Recommendations

Program	Training
PAVE	Scan and flash (numbers and letters) practice
Guided Reading	Timed and scanned directed reading

Figure 8.15

of recognition; improved GPA and visual function tests. (The longer duration of fixation is due to the reduction of fixations and regressions.) While the reading rate was similar to pre-therapy level, there was significant improvement in all binocular vision skills and the patient symptom survey.

Our *Comparison of Multiple Tests* checklist, shown in Figure 8.16, provides instant recognition of this patient's steady improvement throughout the period of vision training. The initial six months of therapy were weekly sessions, whereas the last year was scheduled mainly every three to four weeks. Daily computer-based therapy programs were continued throughout. Patient compliance was more variable during the last six months, which explains some of the changes in rate between the three recordings. Home vision therapy continues with a goal of reducing variability and regression of progress achieved. The data can also be presented in graphs to better illustrate improvements.

VISAGRAPH Results – Comparison of Multiple Tests

Patient Name: TBI therapy patient_ DOB: IEI File #:

	Pre-Vision Therapy	Post-VT #2	Post-VT #3	Comments about Pre & Post Vt results
Visa - Reading	Date: 11/2010	Date: 5/9/11	Date: 6/25/12	(+ = improved; - = worse; ~ no change)
Fix/100wds-L	165	132	107	+ (↓ Fix/100words by 58 fixations)
Fix/100wds-R	166	132	92	+ (↓ Fix/100words by 74 fixations)
Reg/100wds - L	29	14	8	+ (↓ Reg/100words by 21 fixations)
Reg/100wds - R	29	12	10	+ (↓Reg/100words by 19 fixations)
Span(words) L	0.61	0.76	0.93	+ (↑ Span by 0.32 words)
Span(words) R	0.60	0.76	1.09	+ (↑ Span by 0.49 words)
AvDurFix (sec) - L	0.23	0.21	0.32	~
AvDurFix (sec) - R	0.23	0.21	0.37	~
Duration SD	78	98	253	~
Rate - w/min	158	214	176	+ (↑ Rate by 18 w/min)
RateAdj w/o RR	176	231	176	~
OD/OS correlation	99%	98%	87%	~
SaccStarDif	42	47	34	+ (↓ SaccStartDiff by 8 events)
Anom 1	1	2	17	~
Anom 2	0	2	1	~
Anom 3	0	0	1	~
Sacc/Ret/Sweep	23/10 (2.3)	19/10 (1.9)	16/10 (1.6)	+ (↑ Sacc/Accuracy by 0.7 saccades)
Grade (GPE)	3.4	7.3	7.7	+ (↑ Improved GPE by 4.3 grades)

Figure 8.16

Joseph Sullivan, OD, FCOVD
Wichita, Kansas
316–683–8204

Use of the Visagraph in the Kansas Vision and Reading Study

During the 1998 legislative session, the Kansas Legislature approached the Kansas Optometric Association to conduct a research study on the link between an undetected vision problem and the affect it can have on the reading performance of Kansas students. The purpose of this research project was to identify children with a specific vision condition (convergence insufficiency) that is thought to manifest itself as a reduced ability to read for a normal amount of time. Convergence insufficiency, a difficulty in aiming the eyes together to view objects at a close range, such as words in textbooks, is a visual disorder commonly treated by optometric vision therapy.

Fifty-six third-grade students (all diagnosed with convergence insufficiency) completed this study. The students were randomly divided into two groups. A treatment group (36 subjects) underwent vision therapy with the goal of treating the convergence insufficiency. A control group (27 subjects) did not undergo vision therapy.

For the treatment group, the efficiency of vision therapy was assessed by measuring both visual skills and reading performance prior to and after treatment. For the control group, reading performance was assessed prior to and after a period of roughly six months to account for any differences in aging. Visual performance was assessed by near point visual testing. Measures of reading performance included both objective measures of reading eye movements as recorded by the Visagraph eye movement monitor and a reading test chosen by the Kansas State Board of Education. The Visagraph provided the following measures of reading eye movements: fixations, regressions, span of recognition, and duration of fixation. The Visagraph also estimates the reading grade level.

Data analysis was performed by means of a repeated measures Analysis of Variance, with a between factor of pre-treatment (initial visit) verses post-treatment (final visit) score and a within factor of the individual measures. The treatment group showed a significant change over time in 17 of the 26 analyses (65 percent) while the control group only showed a significant change in 7 of the 26 analyses (27 percent).

The measurements of eye movement during reading showed that treatment subjects had gained more efficient reading skills. The Visagraph revealed that the number of fixations per 100 words was significantly reduced ($p=.04000$) from 215.6 fixations before treatment to 192.2 fixations after treatment. In addition, the average span of recognition was increased from .51 words to .60 words (p=.0089). The number of regressions per 100 words was reduced by 11 words (from 51 regressions before therapy to 40 regressions following therapy (p=.0771). Although this measure was not found to be statistically significant, it is interesting and similar results with larger subject numbers would have produced statistically significant data.

The pretest and posttest Visagraph results, shown in the following images, illustrate that optometric vision therapy improved the signs and symptoms of a visual disorder commonly seen in children. In addition, a highly visual task like reading showed significant improvement following optometric therapy. The results are especially profound considering the relatively small subject pool of this study. The studies' areas of emphasis could not have been evaluated without the use of Visagraph recordings and the areas that they can monitor.

In Figure 8.17, a grade two subject's pretest indicates:

- FRP skills are significantly lower than grade level two norms
- Reading Rate is only 58 words per minute
- Cross Correlation is extremely low suggesting binocular coordination problems.

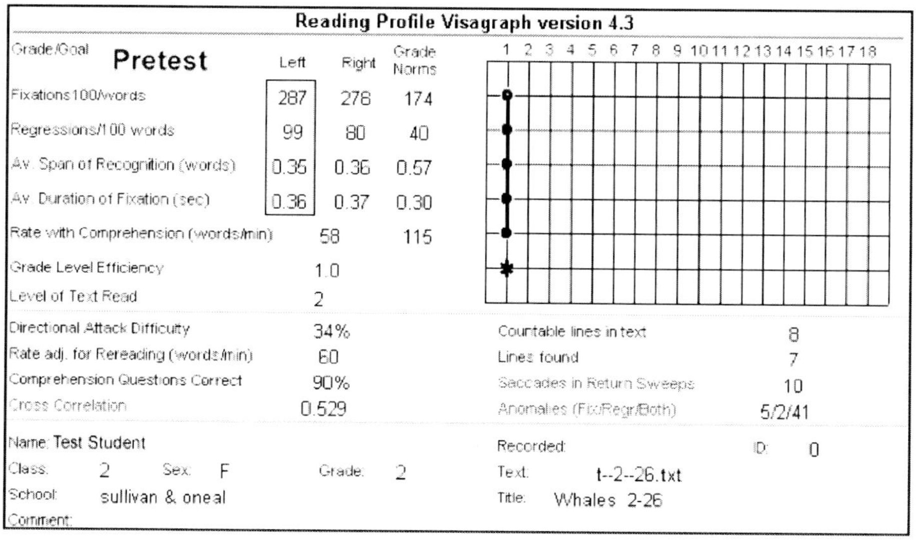

Figure 8.17

In Figure 8.18, the same grade two subject's posttest indicates:

- FRP skills have improved significantly
- Reading Rate is now 106 words per minute
- Cross Correlation, although not as good as might be expected, has improved dramatically.

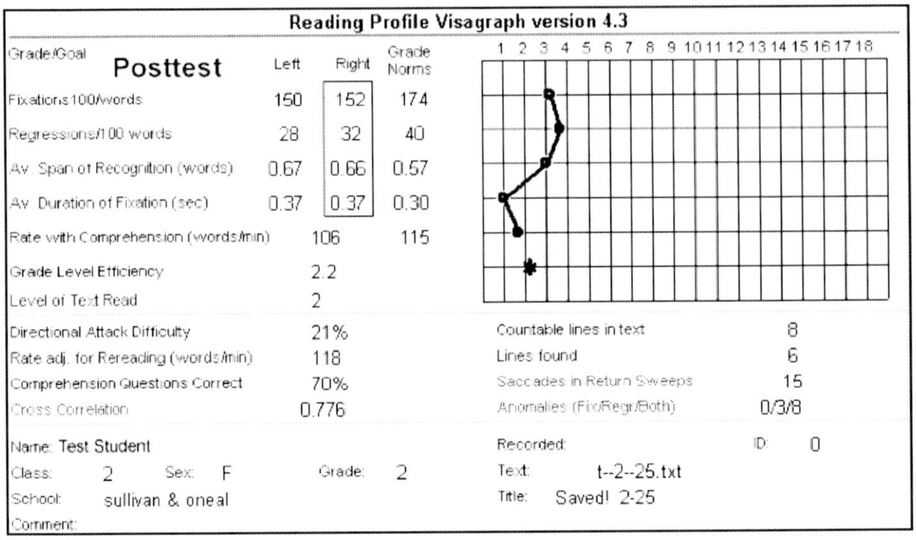

Reading Profile Visagraph version 4.3

Grade/Goal **Posttest**	Left	Right	Grade Norms
Fixations/100 words	150	152	174
Regressions/100 words	28	32	40
Av. Span of Recognition (words)	0.67	0.66	0.57
Av. Duration of Fixation (sec)	0.37	0.37	0.30
Rate with Comprehension (words/min)	106		115
Grade Level Efficiency	2.2		
Level of Text Read	2		

Directional Attack Difficulty	21%	Countable lines in text	8
Rate adj. for Rereading (words/min)	118	Lines found	6
Comprehension Questions Correct	70%	Saccades in Return Sweeps	15
Cross Correlation	0.776	Anomalies (Fix/Regr/Both)	0/3/8

Name: Test Student	Recorded:	ID: 0
Class: 2	Sex: F	Grade: 2	Text: t--2--25.txt
School: sullivan & oneal	Title: Saved! 2-25
Comment:

Figure 8.18

In Figure 8.19, a grade three subject's pretest indicates:

- FRP skills are far lower than grade level three norms
- Reading Rate is only 69 words per minute
- Cross Correlation is extremely low suggesting binocular coordination problems.

In Figure 8.20, the same grade three subject's posttest indicates:

- FRP skills have improved considerably
- Reading Rate is now 114 words per minute
- Cross Correlation is very close to being acceptable.

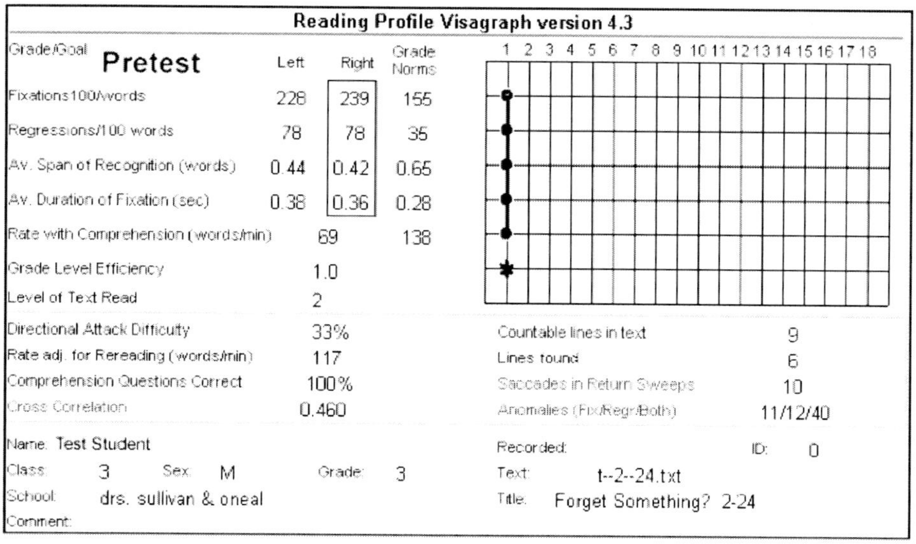

Reading Profile Visagraph version 4.3

Grade/Goal **Pretest**	Left	Right	Grade Norms
Fixations 100/words	228	239	155
Regressions/100 words	78	78	35
Av. Span of Recognition (words)	0.44	0.42	0.65
Av. Duration of Fixation (sec)	0.38	0.36	0.28
Rate with Comprehension (words/min)	69		138
Grade Level Efficiency	1.0		
Level of Text Read	2		

Directional Attack Difficulty	33%	Countable lines in text	9
Rate adj. for Rereading (words/min)	117	Lines found	6
Comprehension Questions Correct	100%	Saccades in Return Sweeps	10
Cross Correlation	0.460	Anomalies (Fix/Regr/Both)	11/12/40

Name: Test Student | Recorded: | ID: 0
Class: 3 | Sex: M | Grade: 3 | Text: t--2--24.txt
School: drs. sullivan & oneal | Title: Forget Something? 2-24
Comment:

Figure 8.19

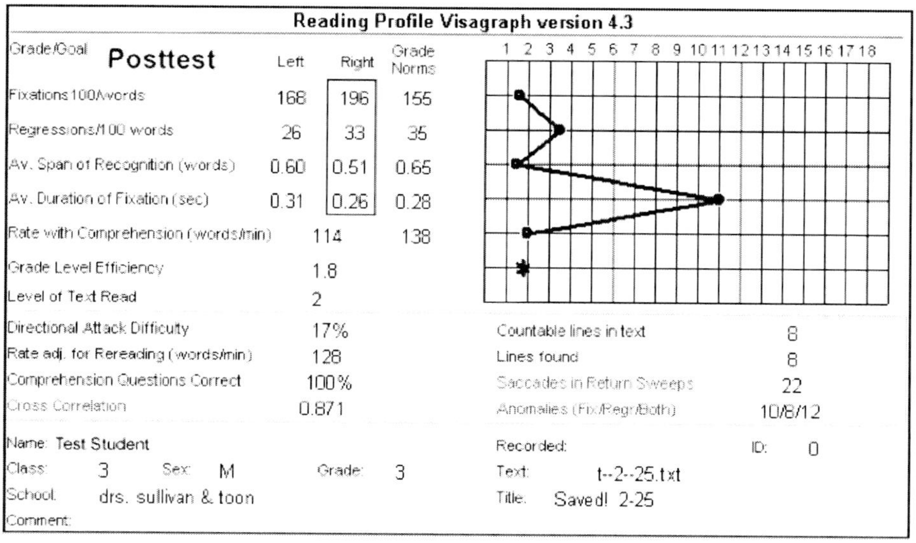

Reading Profile Visagraph version 4.3

Grade/Goal **Posttest**	Left	Right	Grade Norms
Fixations 100/words	168	196	155
Regressions/100 words	26	33	35
Av. Span of Recognition (words)	0.60	0.51	0.65
Av. Duration of Fixation (sec)	0.31	0.26	0.28
Rate with Comprehension (words/min)	114		138
Grade Level Efficiency	1.8		
Level of Text Read	2		

Directional Attack Difficulty	17%	Countable lines in text	8
Rate adj. for Rereading (words/min)	128	Lines found	8
Comprehension Questions Correct	100%	Saccades in Return Sweeps	22
Cross Correlation	0.871	Anomalies (Fix/Regr/Both)	10/8/12

Name: Test Student | Recorded: | ID: 0
Class: 3 | Sex: M | Grade: 3 | Text: t--2--25.txt
School: drs. sullivan & toon | Title: Saved! 2-25
Comment:

Figure 8.20

John A. Thomas, MS, OD, FCOVD, DP
Neuro-Optometric Rehabilitation
Diplomate, American Board of Disability Analysts
Professor, Adjunct, Pacific University College of Optometry
Wheat Ridge, Colorado
V/M: 303-421-4465
FX: 303-431-6771
brainjt@aol.com

I have owned/used at least three evolutions of the valuable and indispensable Visagraph. My OD specialty tract at university was binocular visual function to include specifically strabismus, amblyopia, perception, learning dysfunction, and with Super Clinic, under the direction of the late Dr. William Ludlam–electro diagnostics, specifically VECP, EEG, ERG, EOG, ECG, and dark adaptation analysis. Further, I was a participant in the Neuro Ophthalmological Residency program under the direction of Dr. Neil Barmack, Neuro Sciences Research Center, Portland, Oregon, for a period of three years.

My career as an optometrist has specialized in the diagnosis and treatment of neurological problems affecting the visual function, the entire spectrum from congenital/genetic to acquired. I am co-founder of Neuro Optometric Rehabilitation Association, Int. (NORA), with worldwide membership. We have created the specialty discipline of neuro optometry and have established this discipline in the refereed *Current Eye & Vision Science Literature.* I personally have multiple publications in medical literature. Through our CE, clinical training, and fellowship programs, we have created the largest population of hospital-based optometrists in the profession (the Neuro Optometrist), providing neuro optometric rehabilitation.

Traumatic brain injury (TBI) has been my primary professional pursuit for the whole of my career. My pediatric optometric training was a perfect preparation for this immensely interesting and challenging work. All TBI cases include some degree of oculomotor dysfunction, therefore binocular dysfunction, binocular visual information processing dysfunction(BVIP), and degradation of executive function (EF).

The Visagraph Eye Movement Recording System is the most efficient and cost-effective clinical instrumentation for the diagnostic support, and follow-up, of eye-movement disorders of any etiology. This technology provides objective quantitative analysis with graphic presentation of the patient's eye movements, normative scoring of:

- Fixations/100 words
- Regressions/100 words
- Average Span of Recognition (words)
- Average Duration of Fixation (sec)
- Rate with Comprehension (words/min)
- Grade Level Efficiency
- Level of Text Read

- Directional Attack Difficulty
- Rate Adjusted for Rereading (words per minute)
- Comprehension Questions Correct
- Cross Correlation
- Countable Lines of Text
- Countable Lines of Print Read
- Saccades in Return Sweeps
- Anomalies (Fixations/Regressions/Both)

Computer recording and analysis of the above reading biomechanics (oculo-motor components of the reading eye-movement process) are presented in quantitative form and compared to norms; graphical presentation providing a performance profile rated against academic-year level attained at time of evaluation. Very impressive visual presentation provides a summation of complex data derived from the most sophisticated motor function of *Homo sapiens* in a comprehensive format that is easily and immediately comprehensible to patient, other caregivers, and case managers.

The paragraphs below are characteristic of statement/information that I provide in my IME reports. My records and reports have survived the "crucible" of the courtroom cross-examination in more than 100 "expert witness" testimonies that I have provided. No opposing expert has ever been able, or lacked the knowledge/courage, to deny the efficacy of my reports, especially the Visagraph component.

In my opinion, Taylor Associates has provided the vision care community with instrumentation that is the most effective and cost efficient for the diagnostic support of eye-movement dysfunction. No optometric office is complete without this instrumentation. I have made this statement hundreds of times in my worldwide lectures on every continent regarding TBI and binocular dysfunction. There is no other clinical tool that so supports the optometric services of vision therapy. I have championed the supplanting of VT with binocular visual rehabilitation. The entire medical community, including insurance, recognizes the term and concept of rehabilitation.

Visagraph (photoelectric infrared oculography) is a real-time, task-rated, eye-movement monitoring system that precisely records oculomotor performance under sustained task demand. Performance is graded against established age/grade norms. I include the analytical computer printout and graphs that document this performance; they will be found in the report addendum. The raw data is very voluminous and detailed, and remains on file here in this clinic. Real-time sustained task-demand oculography (eye movement measurement and recording while performing a reading task) provides an objective methodology for demonstrating the patient's ability to perform the highly integrated complex binocular task of reading (eye-movement biomechanics of the reading process).

Additionally, this technology provides an objective method for determining rehabilitative progress. The generalized subjective testing performed by the general vision care provider yields soft, opinion-based qualification of outcome. Instrumentation, such as the Visagraph, VIPS battery, and Campimetry analysis, now exists to provide the scientifically-based, statistically accurate normative, analyzed and graphically output to judge quality of binocular performance objectively, relative to rehabilitation. Such objective analysis brings reliable data to the case manager, enabling sound and confirmable judgments as to achievement of rehabilitative programs and a sound objective basis for assisting with the determination of maximum medical improvement (MMI).

Lynn F. Hellerstein, OD, FAAO, FCOVD
Hellerstein and Brenner Vision Center, P.C.
Centennial, Colorado
303–850–9499
LHellerstein@HBVision.net
www.HBVision.net
www.LynnHellerstein.com

We use the Visagraph test on almost every patient referred to our office for learning/reading problems as long as the patient can read at the second grade level or higher. We test approximately six patients per week.

We repeat Visagraph testing on most of these same vision therapy patients every eight weeks during their vision therapy and at the end of vision therapy.

We use Reading Plus fluency development with some patients along with our optometric vision therapy program. Most of the patients are wearing reading glasses. We see improvements in Visagraph patients who have not used Reading Plus as well as patients who have used

Reading Plus. Also I should mention that we don't use all the instructional modules of Reading Plus as a school would.

Some of our patients show years of growth in silent reading fluency and many of the other measurements displayed by the Visagraph. The percentage varies since we see patients of all ages with, a variety of types of visual problems . . . a diverse group.

Below are some of the pretest and posttest Visagraph results of several of our patients in our vision therapy program.

In Figure 8.21, a grade one subject's pretest indicates:

- All FRP skills are close to grade level one norm behavior
- Reading Rate is only 68 words per minute
- Grade Level Efficiency is only 1.0
- Cross Correlation is 77 percent, which is low.

In Figure 8.22, the same grade one subject's posttest indicates:

- FRP skills are now better than grade level one norms
- Reading Rate has advanced to 125 words per minute with some rereading (130 words per minute with rereading deleted)
- Grade Level Efficiency is 3.1
- Cross Correlation is now 90 percent, acceptable.

In Figure 8.23, a grade four subject's pretest indicates:

- Many FRP skills are well below grade level four norms
- Reading Rate is 130 words per minute
- Grade Level Efficiency is 2.7.

In Figure 8.24, the same grade four subject's posttest indicates:

- All FRP skills are considerably better than expected in relation to grade level four norms
- Reading Rate is now 214 words per minute with slight rereading (231 words per minute with rereading deleted)
- Grade Level Efficiency is now 7.9.

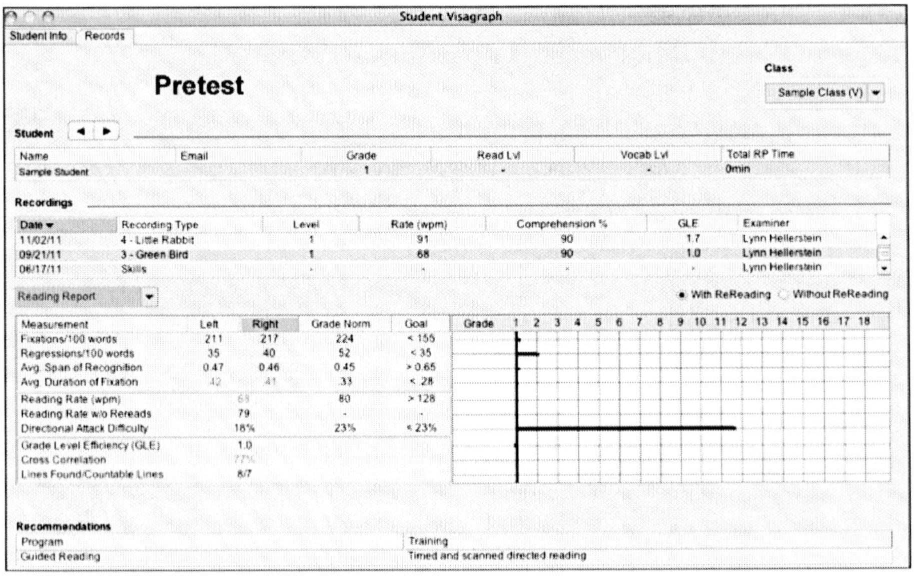

Figure 8.21

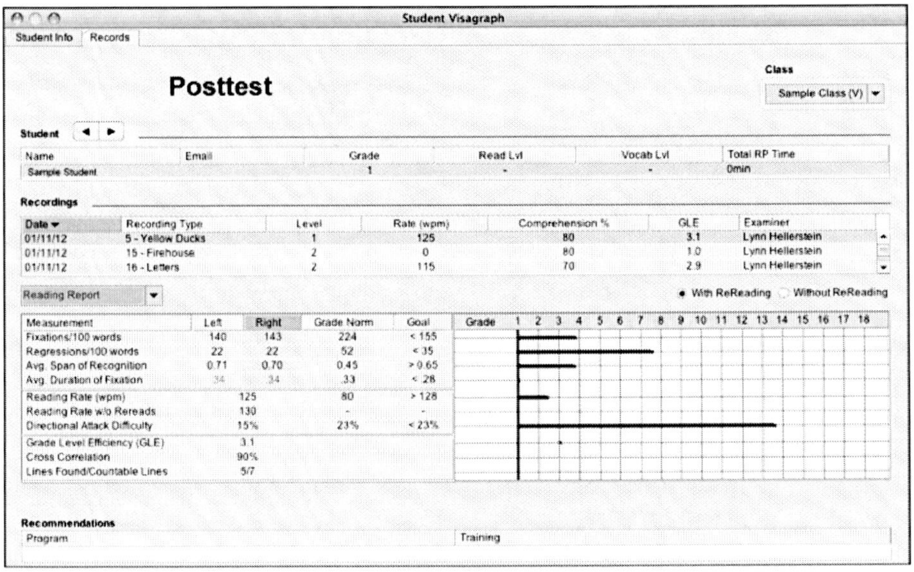

Figure 8.22

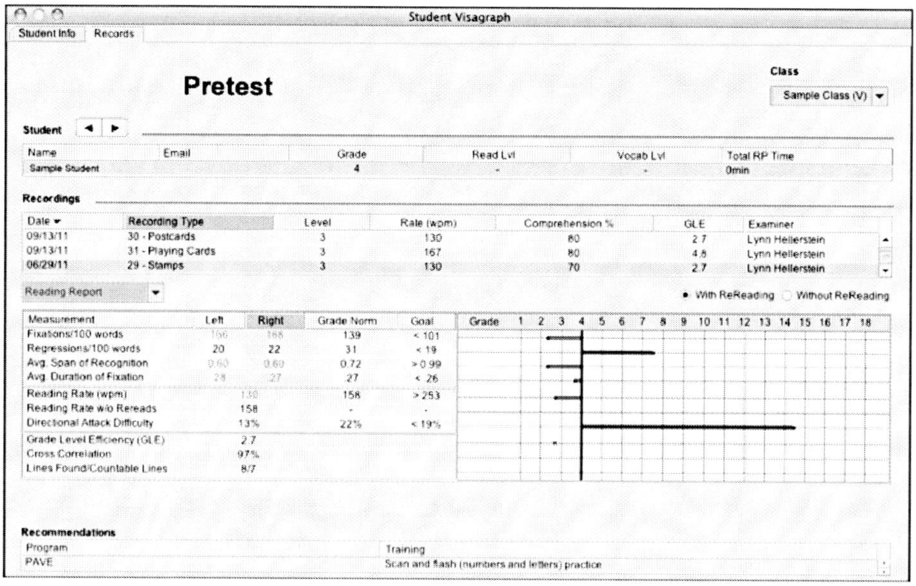

Figure 8.23

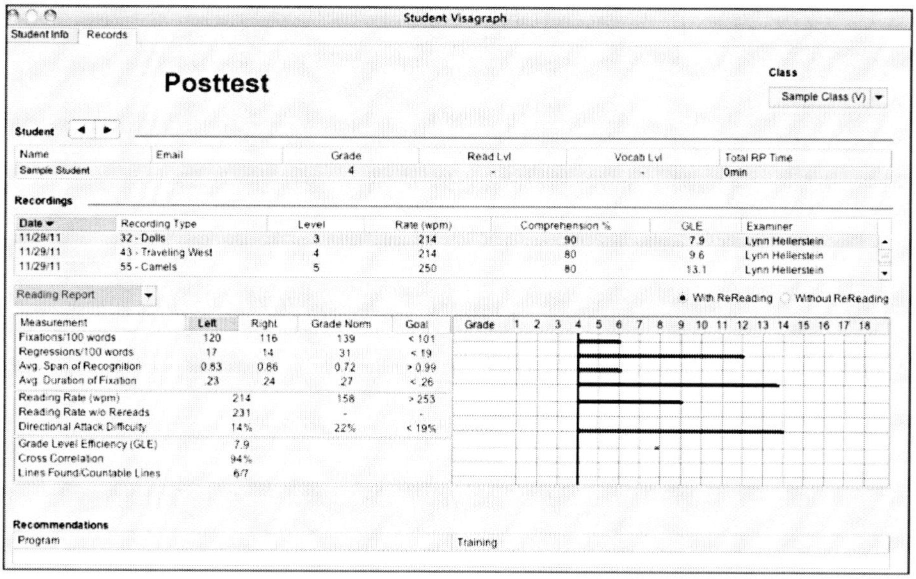

Figure 8.24

In Figure 8.25, a grade five subject's pretest indicates:

- Several FRP skills are lower in performance than grade level five norms
- Reading Rate is only 154 words per minute with some rereading
- Grade Level Efficiency is 4.2
- Cross Correlation is 95 percent, okay.

In Figure 8.26, the same grade five subject's posttest indicates:

- All FRP skills are now considerably better than grade level five norm performance
- Reading Rate is now 231 words per minute with some rereading (273 words per minute with rereading deleted)
- Grade Level Efficiency has advanced to level 10.3
- Cross Correlation is 98 percent.

In Figure 8.27, a grade six subject's pretest indicates:

- Most FRP skills are lower than expected in relation to grade level six norms
- Reading Rate is only 167 words per minute with some rereading
- Grade Level Efficiency is 4.6
- Cross Correlation is 88 percent (suspect).

In Figure 8.28, the same grade six subject's posttest indicates:

- All FRP skills are now very close to grade level six norms
- Reading Rate is now 231 words per minute without rereading
- Grade Level Efficiency is now 7.9
- Cross Correlation has improved to 97 percent.

Alan P Pearson, OD, MEd, PhD, FCOVD
Vision Clinics of Development and Learning
Bothell, Washington
425–213–1016
800–410–1356
appod@askdrpearson.com
www.askdrpearson.com

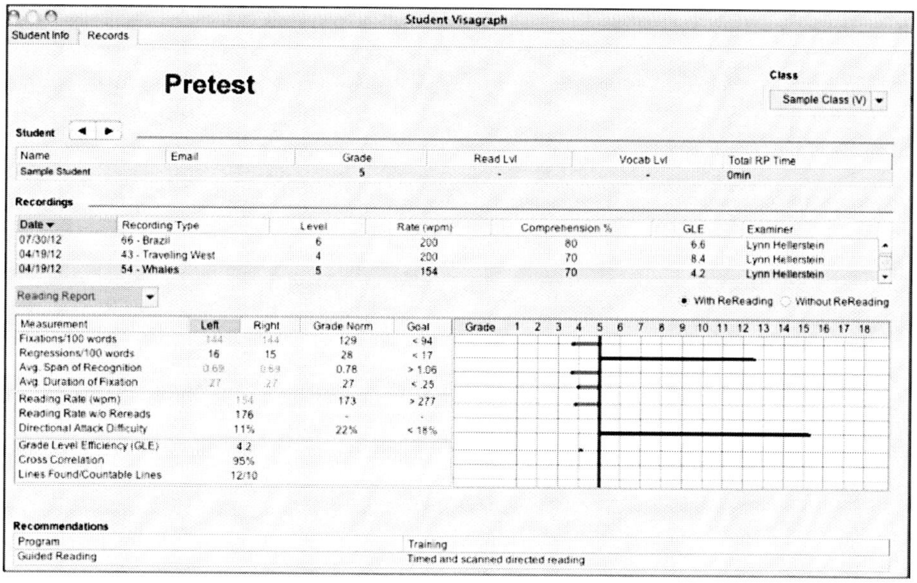

Figure 8.25

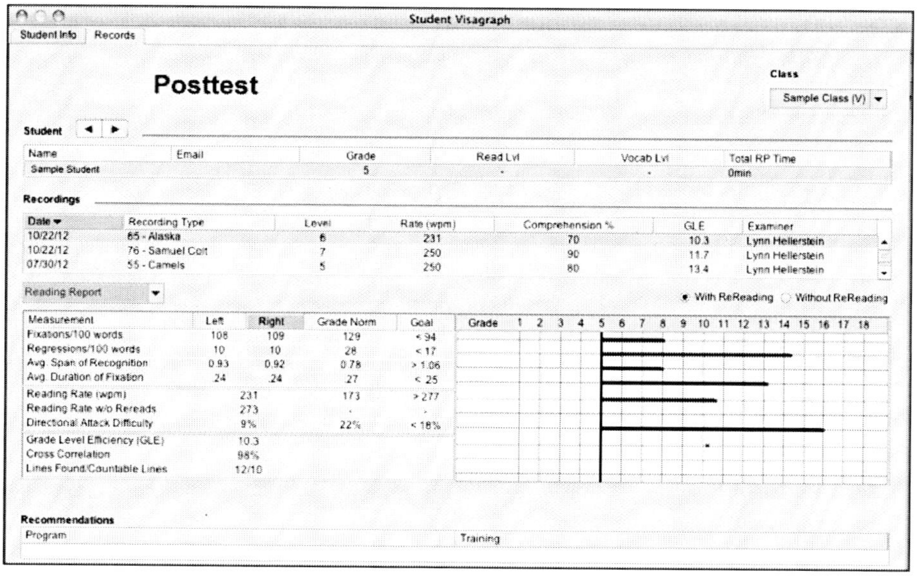

Figure 8.26

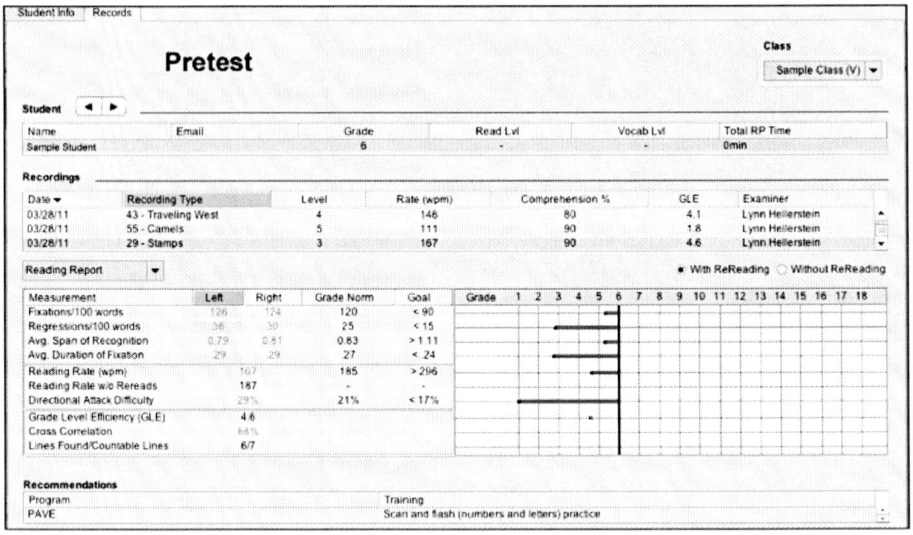

Figure 8.27

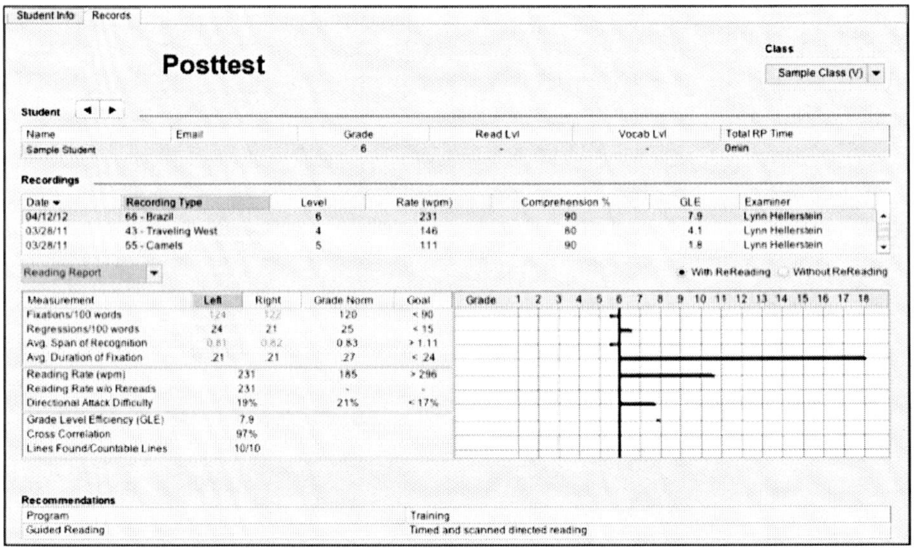

Figure 8.28

When a school-aged patient comes to a vision specialist, such as an optometrist, with a complaint of difficulties related to reading, then tests of visual function that go beyond the standard vision evaluation covering eye health and eye optics are warranted. Before describing some of these functional tests, it is good to step back and consider how the visual system is involved in the reading process. When parents bring their child to my clinic and need to understand what I have found in my evaluation, I usually start with a simple analogy. I describe the visual system as being much like the arm and hand exploring the world.

If you are going to explore with your arm and hand, the first step is to grab hold of the object. This involves the big muscles (gross motor) of the arm that brings the hand in the vicinity of the object, and then the fine motor muscles of the hand and finger that actually grab the object. Feeling the object, which is the meaning and understanding-gathering step, can only occur if the object is in the grasp and being touched and manipulated. Vision is just like this. The first step is to visually grab hold of the object being looked at. This involves big muscles of the body and neck that orient the eyes toward the object, and then fine motor muscles around the eyes to precisely point the eyes at the object. These fine motor movements can be horizontal/vertical for precise orientation or convergence/divergence for the precise binocular vision coordination at the appropriate distance the object is from the eyes. Visual grab also involves the focusing system composed of a muscle and lens just behind the pupil. This focusing (accommodative) system is usually relaxed for the distance and contracts for focusing at near point. When looking at an object the muscle and lens must be precisely used to focus the object at the appropriate distance from the eyes. So, visual grab involves orientation, coordination, and focus, and these abilities need to function in an efficient integrated manner for the next step to occur well.

The next step is visual feel of the object. This is the perceptual and cognitive processing that takes place to gather meaning from the object that is in visual grasp. Perceptual and cognitive processing is impacted by the quality of the visual grasp in a similar way that it is hard to feel an object with the hand if one cannot keep it in the hand's grasp.

Finally, after meaning has been gathered from the object being looked at, then it is time to move the eyes to the next object and repeat the process. The visual system makes jumping eye movements called saccades to move the eyes from one object to another. So if you can imagine a person looking at a picture on the wall, the eyes are involved in a sequence visual grab, jump grab, jump, grab. Or in more detail, what is happening is visual coordination, focus, feel, jump repeated over and over.

Now a picture on the wall doesn't require much order and sequence in this process of viewing; the longer the picture is looked at, the more the eyes jump around gathering meaning. In the process of reading, however, order and sequence is very important. The objects for the eyes to grab are word chunks, which can be pieces of words, whole words, or more than one word. As we become better readers, we are able to pick up bigger chunks with each visual grab (fixation). Then we need to have rapid processing of the words (grapheme) to meaning (phonemes and language). This all has to happen in a fraction of a second. Then we jump our eyes to the next word chunk with a saccade and repeat the grab and feel. This alternation between grab, feel, jump, repeats across the line of print sequentially, and then a large saccade occurs to jump the eyes back to the beginning of the next line. The sequence, order, and patterning of these movements is important for overall reading fluency and comprehension.

With this background, we can now review the important functional tests of vision in the reading process.

1. *Visual Grab:* Visual efficiency factors such as binocular and accommodative interactions will impact the child's abilities to visually grab hold of word chunks. Doctors of optometry have special batteries of assessment tools to assess binocular and accommodative interactions.
2. *Visual Feel:* Visual processing factors such as the ability to rapidly decode word chunks impacts the ability for the child to gather meaning in the short duration of fixation. Optometrists may use assessment tools such as the Developmental Eye Movement Test to probe for automaticity issues. There are many psychoeducational tests of reading that will probe processing issues.
3. *Visual Jump:* Saccadic praxis, or the ability to move the eyes in an organized and efficient left-to-right, top-to-bottom fashion impacts the child's overall reading fluency and comprehension. The Developmental Eye Movement Test probes saccadic eye tracking in a context similar to reading and helps to differentiate between auto-

matic processing and saccadic tracking difficulties. To really understand how saccadic praxis is developing within the context of silent reading, infrared eye tracking during the reading process is necessary. The Visagraph is a device that does this and also provides additional clues to the evaluator about the child's visual grab and visual feel of word chunks. The Visagraph is an essential tool in a comprehensive evaluation of vision in the reading process.

I do a routine Visagraph test on all grade-school-age children. In my experience, those who complete a program of vision therapy do not always show significant improvements in their Visagraph Reading Reports. For these individuals, I then recommend Reading Plus. I ask them to complete 100 or more stories in the four-month period (60 to 80 sessions is more common). Following the use of Reading Plus, the Visagraph results are always much improved.

I use my Visagraph with every school-age patient I see. I currently work in a multidisciplinary setting along with occupational therapy, speech-language pathology, and physical therapy. A lot of my patients are preschool, but I do have a fair number of grade school patients, too. I only do functional vision assessments currently. I also provide vision therapy services. I have a three-phase approach to reading struggles:

1. I work with the binocular vision issues, such as convergence insufficiency, first. Then when visual grab is functioning well, I start integrating the visual skill into reading processing.
2. I have a course of treatment I call Foundations that works on decoding and processing skills. I use Lexia Reading as a core component of this course.
3. When binocular and processing are functioning well I move the patient to the Fluency course, which uses Reading Plus as the core software.

Theodore S. Kadet, OD, FCOVD
Developmental Vision Associates, PLLC/dba Hope Clinic
Bellevue, Washington
Phone: 425–462–7800
FAX: 425–455–3019
tsk@hopecliniconline.com
www.hopecliniconline.com

I have a practice limited to developmental and neuro-optometry. I do no primary care. I see two main patient populations. My typical patient is an eight- to 15-year-old student, smart, but achieving below potential in school (typical binocular dysfunction issues). The other major area is neuro-optometry–patients with vision dysfunctions from a closed-head injury, or traumatic brain injury.

Visagraph tests are administered to every patient who can fluently read material at the first grade reading level or higher. This is a standard part of my vision evaluation as it is the most powerful tool I have to demonstrate vision problems to parents/patients. I give the patient a copy of the Visagraph results to take home, along with my explanation summary for other parent/family members, etc. to review.

In Figure 8.29, a grade four subject's pretest indicates:

- Most FRP skills are lower than grade level four norms (number of Fixations per 100 word selection)
- Reading Rate is 176 words per minute (slightly higher than grade four norms)
- Grade Level Efficiency is only 2.7
- Cross Correlation is 88 percent (lower than 90 percent and cause for alarm).

In Figure 8.30, the same grade four subject's posttest indicates:

- FRP skills are now at or above grade level four norms
- Reading Rate has advanced to 300 words per minute without rereading
- Grade Level Efficiency (GLE) is 14.0
- Cross Correlation is now improved to 99 percent.

In Figure 8.31, a grade four subject's pretest indicates:

- Fixations per 100 words is slightly lower than grade level four norms
- Reading Rate is 158 words per minute without rereading
- Grade Level Efficiency is 4.7 (close to grade level norms)
- Cross Correlation is okay.

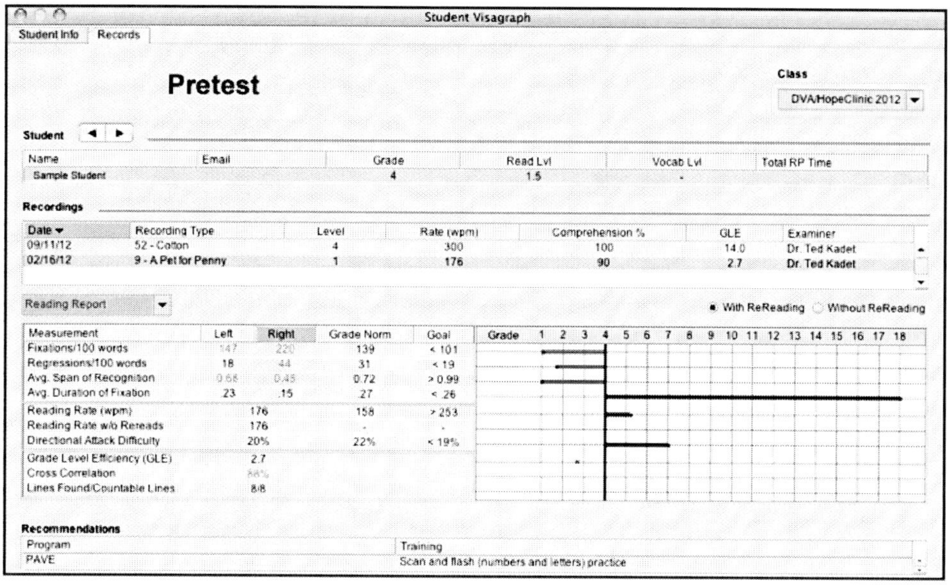

Figure 8.29

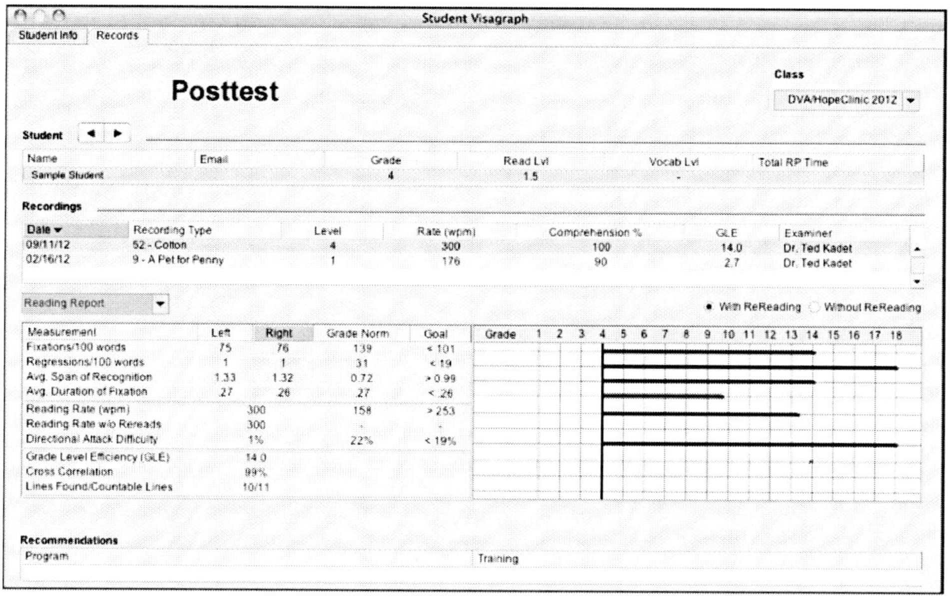

Figure 8.30

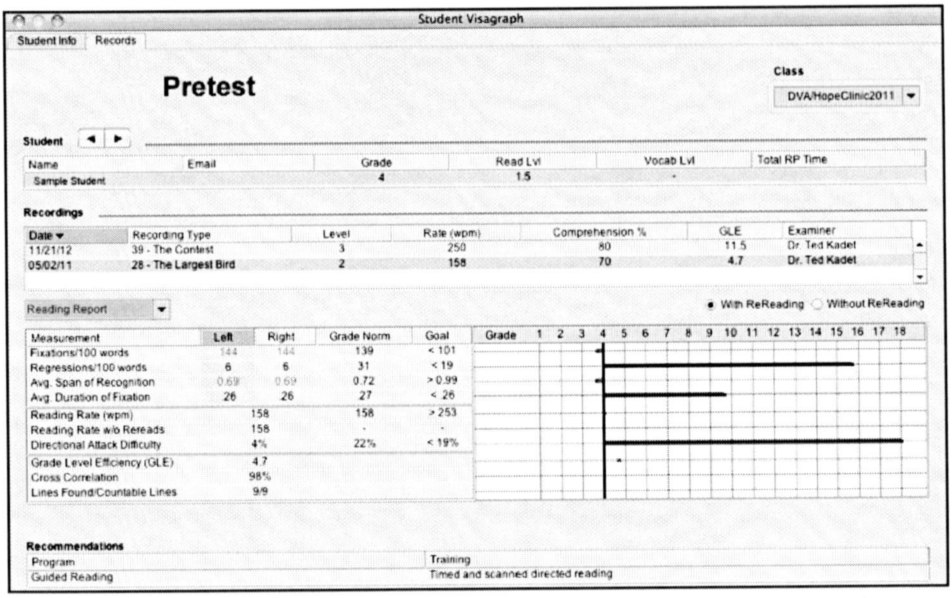

Figure 8.31

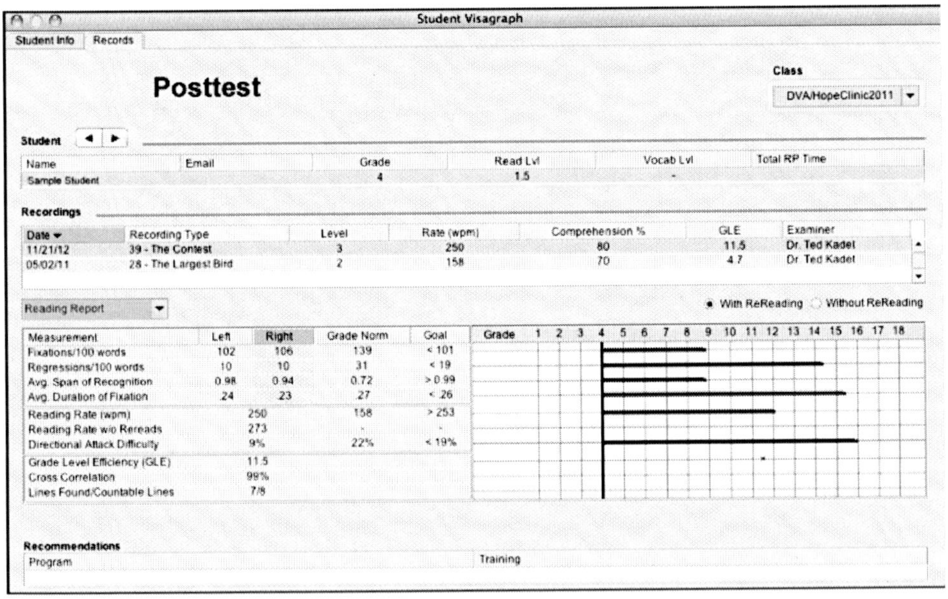

Figure 8.32

In Figure 8.32, the same grade four subject's posttest indicates:

- All FRP skills are better than expected for grade level four
- Reading Rate is now 250 words per minute with slight rereading (271 words per minute with rereading deleted)
- Grade Level Efficiency is now 11.5
- Cross Correlation is okay.

In Figure 8.33, a grade six subject's pretest indicates:

- FRP skills are lower than grade level six norms; however, Fixations per 100 words is higher than expected
- Reading Rate is only 130 words per minute
- Grade Level Efficiency is only 2.6
- Cross Correlation is okay.

In Figure 8.34, the same grade six subject's posttest indicates:

- All FRP skills are now at or slightly higher than grade level six norms
- Reading Rate is now 300 words per minute without rereading
- Grade Level Efficiency is now 13.5
- Cross Correlation is okay.

In Figure 8.35, a college-level subject's pretest indicates:

- Fixations per 100 words is slightly higher than college level norms
- Reading Rate is 273 words per minute with some rereading (286 words per minute with rereading deleted)
- Grade Level Efficiency is 12.7
- Cross Correlation is okay.

In Figure 8.36, the same college-level subject's posttest indicates:

- FRP skills are up to college level norms or above
- Reading Rate is only 400 words per minute without rereading
- Grade Level Efficiency is now 14.9 (advanced level).

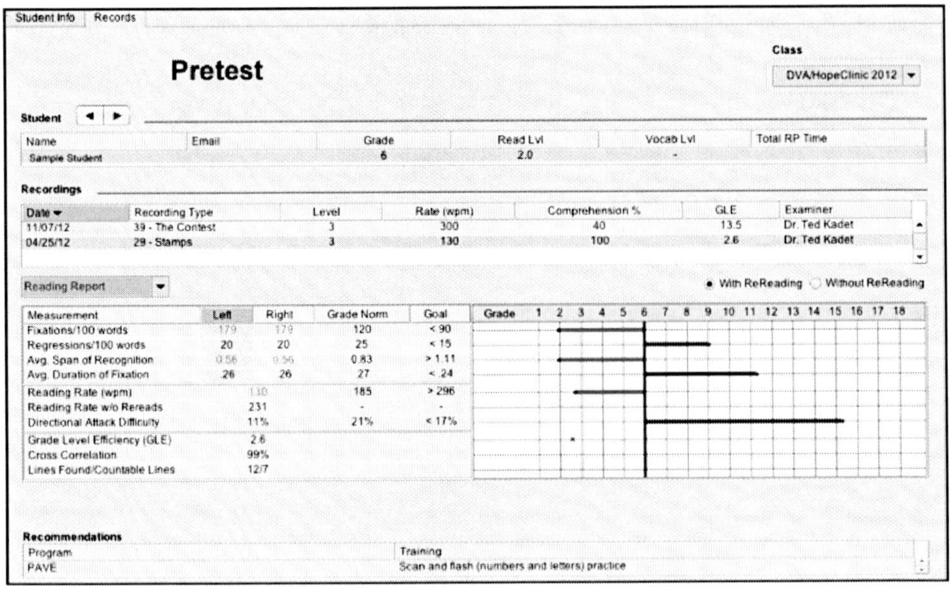

Figure 8.33

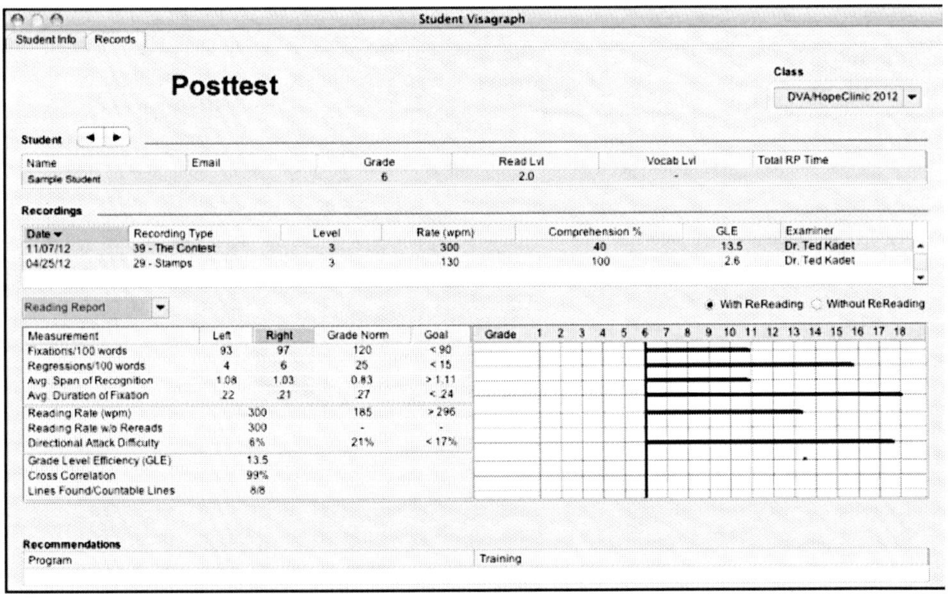

Figure 8.34

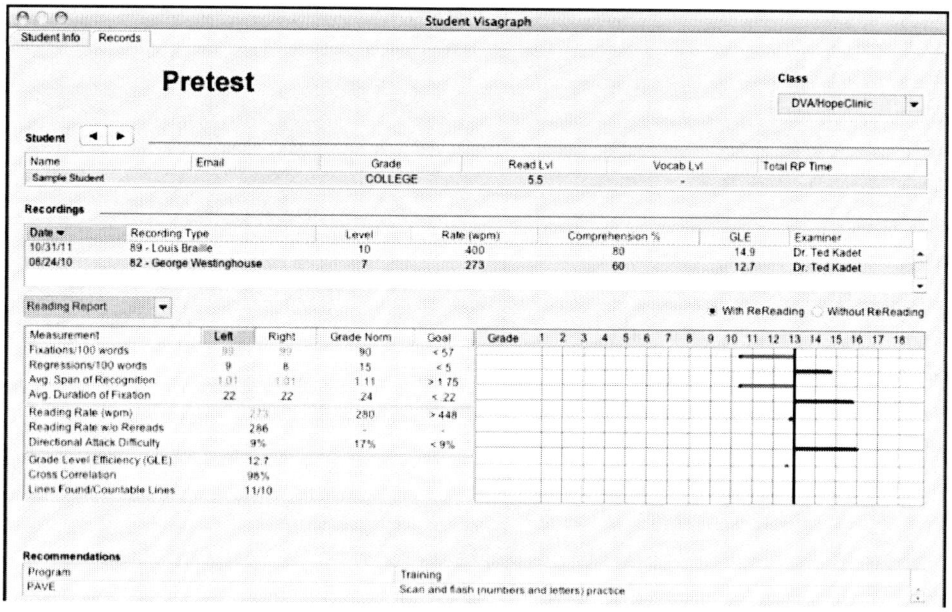

Figure 8.35

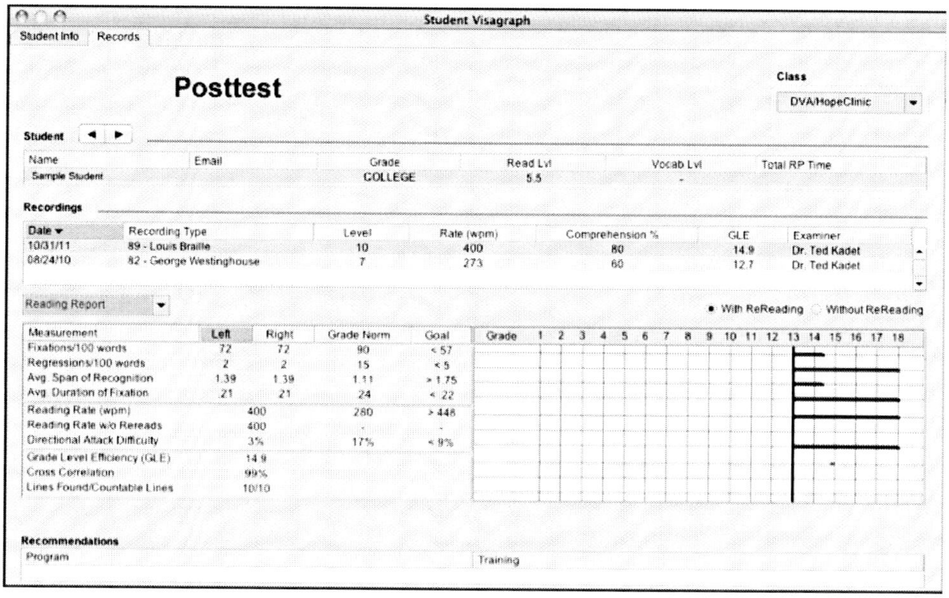

Figure 8.36

CONCLUSION

Eye-movement recording is an invaluable measure of reading performance efficiency and is being used by thousands of schools, clinics, and optometrists. It is primarily used to document changes in the Fundamental Reading Process in terms of changes in a reader's number of fixations, regressions, increased span of recognition, decreases in duration of fixation time, increase in rates of reading, and improvement in visual/functional skills. It is essential that every student at any stage of reading development be at or above the grade level norms specified as appropriate for his or her grade level.

QUESTIONS THAT COULD ARISE AFTER READING THIS CHAPTER

1. In relation to your instructional setting, how might eye-movement recording be incorporated into your diagnostic routine as an effective measure of reading-performance efficiency, and what goals might you set for each student engaged in your visual training activities?
2. How can Visagraph findings in schools result in referrals to your clinic or visual training?
3. What are the results of your vision training program in relation to reading performance, as well as visual/functional efficiency?
4. How might reading fluency development practice, such as Reading Plus, be incorporated into your vision training routine, especially as home-study lessons?
5. How do you evaluate the ease and comfort during reading after vision training and possibly reading-fluency development?

Chapter 9

2010 NORM STUDY USING THE VISAGRAPH EYE MOVEMENT RECORDING SYSTEM

This chapter describes a pilot study conducted by the Research Department of Taylor Associates/Communications (in Winooski, VT) in 2010.

During 2010, a total of 2,196 public school students were tested with the Visagraph III Eye Movement Recording System to see how today's eye movement norms compare with the original eye movement recording study conducted by this author in the 1960s with the Reading Eye II camera. Students in this study were tested only in grades two, four, six, eight, 10, and 12 on the assumption that the data from these even grades would serve as benchmarks to estimate mid-range performance for the odd grades. Each student was first tested on a below grade level selection, for the most part two readability levels lower than grade level, while reading two additional selections on grade level.

A total of 34 schools participated in this 2010 study. The distribution of student numbers across participating states and cities is listed in Table 9.1 follows.

Table 9.1

2010 Taylor Norms							
		Number of Students by Grade					
State	**City**	**2**	**4**	**6**	**8**	**10**	**12**
AR	Jonesboro	29		30			
AR	Lake Village		59			16	13
CA	Gardena	50	45				
CO	Castle Rock	89				64	55
CO	Fort Morgan					31	24
CO	Parker			86	91		
CT	Old Saybrook			30	30		
FL	Tallahassee	30	35				
KS	Kingman	42	48				
LA	Boutte	16	15	10			
LA	Metairie		30				
MA	Athol			23	26		
MA	Lawrence			40	46		
MO	Kirkwood	56	57				
MO	Naylor	26				32	
MO	Portageville				50	55	
MO	St. Louis		49			11	68
MO	Van Buren				27	35	30
NH	Manchester	21	20				
MJ	Hazlet						27
NJ	Parlin		48				
NM	Carlsbad			35	27	30	25
OH	Cambridge	34					
OH	Cleveland			47			
OH	Marysville				84		
SD	Belle Fourche			17	45		
TX	Mission	42	46	1			
VT	Williston				48		
TOTALS		**435**	**452**	**319**	**474**	**274**	**242**

The findings of this preliminary norm study in terms of reading rate are shown in Table 9.2. As you can see, the findings of the 2010 study compared with the 1960 ReadingEye norm study rates show that students in grade two were close to the rate performance in the 1960 study. However, reading rate performances for grades four, six, eight, 10, and 12 were substantially lower and these performances between the 1960 and 2010 study decreased steadily from grades four through 12.

Table 9.2

Taylor Norms						
Average Reading Rate (wpm) of all Recordings with ≥ 70% Comprehension	**Grade**					
	2	**4**	**6**	**8**	**10**	**12**
1960 Norms	115.0	158.0	185.0	204.0	224.0	250.0
2010 Grade Level Tests	116.4	154.0	164.2	165.2	178.7	195.4

Note in Table 9.3 of students in grades two through 12 that the number of fixations per 100 words was also higher than the 1960 norm performance in all grades indicating less fluent reading.

Table 9.3

Taylor Norms						
Average Fixations of all Recordings with ≥ 70% Comprehension	**Grade**					
	2	**4**	**6**	**8**	**10**	**12**
1960 Norms	174.0	139.0	120.0	109.0	101.0	94.0
2010 Grade Level Tests	190.1	148.0	143.2	148.9	136.9	131.9

Note in Table 9.4 that the number of regressions at grade level two through six was significantly less than the 1960 norm performance whereas the number of regressions in grades 8 through 12 was greater than the 1960 study.

Table 9.4

Taylor Norms						
Average Regressions of all Recordings with ≥ 70% Comprehension	Grade					
	2	4	6	8	10	12
1960 Norms	40.0	31.0	25.0	21.0	19.0	17.0
2010 Grade Level Tests	32.8	26.7	23.4	26.7	21.3	21.1

During the initial testing process, each student was tested two levels below his or her grade level. However, grade two students were tested on a grade one level reading selection. Following this, all students read four selections at their grade level.

The reason for testing students below grade level was to determine whether they had the ability to read more fluently on easier content. Additionally, the reason for having each student read four selections at their grade level was to be sure that all students had the opportunity to show their consistent level of silent reading fluency. In the 1960 study, the number of students was approximately 1,000 per grade level and from this more limited study sufficient data was needed to be sure of the fluency benchmarks for the even grades.

Interestingly, the reading rates of students reading a test selection two levels below grade level (with the exception of grade two in which students read a selection one level lower) with 70 percent or higher comprehension did not display a higher reading rate until grade six and this rate was still not as fluent as the 1960 norm rate, as shown in Table 9.5. Rate of reading today is much slower than in the 1960s. Presumably, this stems from the students' tendency to make more fixations and regressions per 100 words than was shown in the 1960 study. To be explicit, students are reading about 20 percent slower in the 2010 study in relation to the 1960 study and even when students read easier content the reading rates did not reach the 1960 level.

Likewise, students also dropped in the number of fixations in grades six through 12 when reading the easier content, but did not substantially drop below the 1960 norms, as shown in Table 9.6.

However, the number of regressions, except for grade two, did drop to a level lower than the 1960 and the 2010 recordings of grade level content as shown in Table 9.7.

Table 9.5

Taylor Norms						
Average Reading Rate (wpm) of all Recordings with ≥ 70% Comprehension	Grade					
	2	4	6	8	10	12
1960 Norms	115.0	158.0	185.0	204.0	224.0	250.0
2010 Grade Level Tests	116.4	154.0	164.2	165.2	178.7	195.4
2010 Two Levels Below Grade Level*	107.6	147.8	169.9	191.6	189.6	234.0

*Results based on students reading passages two levels below grade level except Grade 2 which is based on Level 1 text.

Table 9.6

Taylor Norms						
Average Fixations of all Recordings with ≥ 70% Comprehension	Grade					
	2	4	6	8	10	12
1960 Norms	174.0	139.0	120.0	109.0	101.0	94.0
2010 Grade Level Tests	190.1	148.0	143.2	148.9	136.9	131.9
2010 Two Levels Below Grade Level*	175.0	148.2	124.0	125.3	123.1	119.7

*Results based on students reading passages two levels below grade level except Grade 2 which is based on Level 1 text.

Table 9.7

Taylor Norms						
Average Regressions of all Recordings with ≥ 70% Comprehension	Grade					
	2	4	6	8	10	12
1960 Norms	40.0	31.0	25.0	21.0	19.0	17.0
2010 Grade Level Tests	32.8	26.7	23.4	26.7	21.3	21.1
2010 Two Levels Below Grade Level*	33.2	23.8	19.8	19.3	16.9	15.8

*Results based on students reading passages two levels below grade level except Grade 2 which is based on Level 1 text.

CONCLUSION

Overall, the findings indicate that students in 2010 were not as fluent, in general, as students in the 1960s, especially in grade six and higher.

Span of recognition, which is a function of the number of fixations employed, used to be about one word by grade 11 in the 1960 norm study. Now the span of recognition is less than one word even at grade 12, displaying an average only .67 of a word. This means that word perception is more limited, and this will undoubtedly affect phrasing and a more limited span of recognition, which will affect the reader's use of the right periphery.

Likewise, regressions are higher for grades eight through 12 reading grade level content, which indicates that input into short-term memory is more random and wandering in nature.

The reason for this drop in reading fluency performance over the years needs further exploration, however, these findings are sufficient to raise the question as to why students are not as fluent in silent reading today, especially in grade six and higher.

Is it possible that the largely whole language nature of core beginning reading programs does not adequately prepare students for meaningful fluency in silent reading? A possible explanation may be the lack of high frequency core vocabulary repetitions in today's basals. More explanation is required, but the study suggests what is needed by students today is a strong silent reading fluency development program such as Reading Plus.

Chapter 10

VISAGRAPH/EYELINK1000 COMPARISON STUDY

The following is a summary of a comparison study that was conducted by Dr. Christian Vorstius and Dr. Ralph Radach at Florida State University in 2010 (in press).

The Visagraph Eye Movement Recording System is a commercially available low-cost eye-tracking device that provides an easy way to assess an individual's silent reading efficiency. The browser-based Visagraph III is the latest in a series of eye-movement recording techniques that originated with the Opthalmograph in the 1930s, the Reading Eye in the 1960s, the Eye Track (Reading Eye II) in the 1970s, the Visagraph I in the 1980s, and the Ober II and Visagraph II in the 1990s.

The Visagraph III uses infrared optics in a goggle-style system to track the border between the iris and the sclera to determine the number of all eye movements. The system was designed for use in applied settings, such as optometry practices, reading clinics, and classroom environments, as an effective reading efficiency and diagnostic screening routine. Its purpose is to measure the most fundamental visuomotor aspects of reading, including fluency of information acquisition and regularity of viewing or scanning behavior.

To conduct a silent reading test, Visagraph goggles are placed over a participant's eyes and adjusted to align with the pupils. Standardized reading material is provided with the system that consists of short grade-level-appropriate paragraphs. After a participant reads a paragraph, a comprehension score is determined using ten true/false questions. Eye movement and comprehension data are automatically analyzed, and reports on the characteristics of a reader's visuomotor activity are saved. The data includes basic parameters, such as number of fixations, fixation duration, as well as reading rate (words per minute), saccade-type classifications (progressive, regressive, rereading, return sweep, blink, artifacts), and binocular coordination variables.

Each of these parameters can be related to specific processing aspects during reading, and they provide users with insight into the efficiency of a participant's silent reading patterns. Individual findings are assessed in relation to normative grade-level data established in a large-scale norm study involving 12,000 students ranging from grades one through college conducted by Taylor et al. (1960).

Results of a Visagraph test may be used to suggest instructional modifications to better meet a student's learning needs, to provide students with a visual representation of "how" they read, and to track short- and long-term reading improvement.

The degree of accuracy and reliability of an eye-tracking device depends heavily on its intended use. Devices used in cutting-edge experimental research require the highest possible spatial and temporal resolution, allowing for near-perfect accuracy and millisecond precision. By contrast, applications in many applied and clinical settings may be well served with more affordable recording systems that provide reliable monitoring of core reading proficiency measures. However, any cost-benefit analysis for a particular field of application (e.g., optometric assessment or visuomotor training) should be based on objective performance data, ideally from studies comparing different systems.

Until now, there had been no scientific study demonstrating the validity and measurement accuracy of the current-generation Visagraph III. Clearly, the best way to accomplish this goal was to directly compare the Visagraph III with the "gold standard" state-of-the-art eye-tracking system, the EyeLink1000 (www.sr-research.com), a highly respected product used in scientific research laboratories around the world.

Vorstius and Radach (in press) tracked participants on the Visagraph and the EyeLink1000 *simultaneously*, allowing for a detailed direct comparison of critical eye-movement parameters.

The results of this study indicate that the Visagraph produces valid reading eye-movement parameters, especially when used to measure reading performance efficiency in silent reading. The most critical conditions are the evaluations of the number of fixations, average duration of fixations, and reading rate. Regressions should be considered but only if rereading is not considered as a regression. The study proved that these parameters, when tested using the Visagraph, compared well to the same parameters obtained with the EyeLink1000. All procedures of the study were approved by the Florida State University Institutional Review Board.

Study Format

The test subjects were 32 introductory psychology students, 14 male, 18 female. Their mean age was 19.4. All were native English speakers and had normal or corrected-to-normal vision.

When using the Visagraph on its own, the reading material is printed on paper, but in this study the reading material was presented on a standard digital setup that enabled concurrent recordings with both the Visagraph and the EyeLink1000. Reading materials consisted of 11 paragraphs with 12 lines each, taken from the Visagraph Test Booklet (selections 87–97). Paragraphs were presented in one of two type formats, referred to as the *native Visagraph* (NVG) format and the *standard experimental* (EXP) format. Each participant was presented with five paragraphs in each format plus one practice paragraph.

The NVG format uses justified text in Times New Roman font, presented at a typical reading viewing distance of 17 inches (43 cm) and corresponding to 16.5 degrees of visual angle per line.

For the EXP format, paragraphs were presented left aligned in non-proportional Courier New font. Paragraphs were presented on a 22-inch CRT monitor, using a screen resolution of 1024 by 768 at a refresh rate of 120Hz. Together with a viewing distance of 65cm, this resulted in a horizontal visual angle of 0.33 degrees per letter and 16.5 degrees of visual angle per line in both the EXP and NVG formats.

The Visagraph is a limbus tracker, using infrared diodes to illuminate the eye to detect the border between the iris and the sclera. The eye position is sampled with 60Hz, and recording is binocular. While the Visagraph records data for both eyes, for the purpose of this study only, the performance of the right eye was compared with the EyeLink.

The Visagraph records and evaluates only horizontal eye movements. Saccadic movements are taken to be significant when the inter fixation distance (mean location of samples) equals or exceeds 2.4 percent of the passage line width in the Visagraph (NVG) presentation format. This translates into the recognition of a saccadic movement when the movement exceeds about .39 degrees, corresponding to one to two letter spaces in the standardized material used. In addition, a velocity criterion is used to differentiate saccades from concurrent head movements.

The EyeLink1000 is a video-based pupil and corneal reflection tracking system (SR Research Ltd.), sampling at 1000Hz. It has a relative spatial resolution in the order of a few minutes of arc and its absolute accuracy is better than 1/3 degree, depending on calibration. A nine-point calibration was performed before each paragraph. Mean average position error in an accuracy validation routine was not to exceed 0.33 degrees of visual angle. The on-line saccade parser of the eye-tracking system was set to detect saccades with an amplitude of 0.15 degrees or greater, using an acceleration threshold of $8000°/sec^2$ and a velocity threshold of 30 degrees per second. These settings have proven to produce highly accurate and reliable data in multiple reading studies across different laboratories.

Study Procedure

For the purpose of this study, participants sat in front of a monitor and read through the instructions for the reading task presented on the monitor in front of them (see Figure 10.1). First, the participants put on and adjusted Visagraph goggles. Next, they put their head onto a chin rest to adjust the EyeLink1000 camera, shown in the following image. Both Visagraph and EyeLink1000 recordings were conducted at the same time. After ensuring that both systems yielded good readings, the EyeLink1000 was calibrated using a nine-point calibration routine.

Following successful calibration, a fixation target appeared, centered at the top of the screen. When detecting a stable fixation on this target, the experimenter started the Visagraph recording that resulted in an auditory signal. This signal triggered the appearance of the text material on the screen and also synchronized the data streams from both the Visagraph and the EyeLink1000 systems.

Participants read the paragraphs at their usual pace of reading so that they would understand the content and could answer 10 true/false

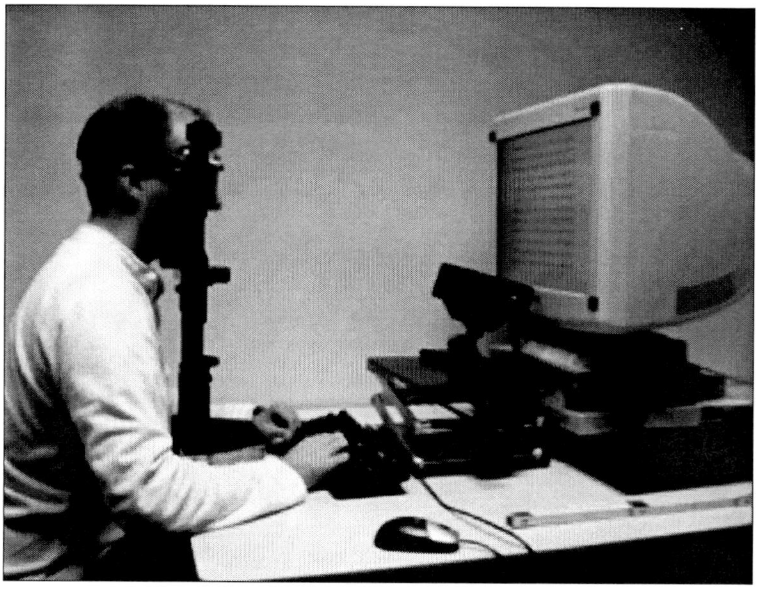

Figure 10.1

comprehension questions when they were done. When finished reading and answering the 10 questions, participants closed their eyes and said, "Done," and the experimenter stopped both recording systems.

Study Results

Eye-movement data from all participants was examined page by page to determine recording quality. For the Visagraph system, an expert inspected the original graph (raw data depiction) visually; for the EyeLink data, standard word-level eye-movement parameters (e.g., fixation duration, gaze duration, total viewing time, initial landing position distribution) were checked in addition to a visual inspection. Pages with poor recording quality or too much missing data in either system were excluded from analyses. Furthermore, only data from participants that produced at least eight passages with acceptable data quality in both systems were used. In all, 30 data sets that included 303 out of 330 test selections were analyzed.

Data from both systems were synchronized and merged into one matrix. Although an auditory signal was used to trigger the start of the text display on the screen, the two devices did not necessarily start at the exact same millisecond. Synchronization adjustments were made, allowing for an optimal level of data aggregation without losing too much information.

For statistical analyses of specific eye-movement parameters, data from the first and last lines within each passage were eliminated. This was necessary because the default data trimming in the integrated Visagraph analyses software uses this algorithm, resulting in the analysis of precisely 100 words per page.

Generally, saccade-type classification matched very well between the two tracking devices with respect to fixations following progressive saccades, blinks, and return sweep parts, but there were differences for fixations following regressive saccades and re-readings. However, these discrepancies are a result of different definitions for re-readings and regressive saccades between the two systems. Taken together, regressive saccades and re-reads account for about 15 percent of the saccades in both EyeLink and Visagraph data, again showing a good match between the two systems.

Examining the critical parameters in more detail, we confirmed that the saccade-type classification matched well between the two systems. The overall slightly higher number of fixations detected in the EyeLink data can be explained with the higher spatial and temporal resolution of this system (1000Hz compared to 60Hz in the Visagraph), leading to the detection of more and shorter fixations. Looking at the percentages for the different saccade types, it is apparent that the classification for progressive saccades, blinks, return sweeps, and return sweep parts is virtually identical between the two eye trackers. The difference between the two systems was fewer than two fixations per typical 100-word recording. However, there were substantial differences in the classifications of regressive saccades and re-readings. This discrepancy can be easily explained by different definitions of "re-reading" in which the Visagraph distinguishes a re-read based on a larger percentage of regressive movement than is typical for a regression. When *re-reading* and *regressions* measures were combined, the difference between EyeLink and Visagraph data almost vanished.

Initially, it appeared that fixation durations within the Visagraph were substantially longer. However, this was related to the fact that within the current Visagraph design, saccade durations are included in the fixation durations. When the Visagraph was adjusted to exclude saccade time, these differences were greatly reduced. Although the exclusion algorithm was rather crude, it confirmed that the underlying approach can be further refined for future iterations of the Visagraph. When, on the other hand, fixation duration and saccade times were combined within the EyeLink, both devices were almost identical.

Both reading rate and "span of recognition" (or number of words processed per fixation) measures were practically identical between the Visagraph and the EyeLink.

Further analysis was conducted to compare fixation duration distribution and line assignment, and although there were variations between the two recording devices, the overall match between the two systems remained consistently good.

Conclusion

The Radach/Vorstius study is the first attempt to validate a widely used low-cost eye-tracking device (Visagraph) against an extremely precise, high-end eye recording system (EyeLink1000). Using both measurement systems simultaneously during data collection enabled a direct comparison of eye-movement parameters in both data streams, allowing a well-grounded assessment on the validity of data collected with the Visagraph system. Given the physical restrains due to the simultaneous tracking setup, which might have prevented optimal Visagraph setup in some cases, the results represent conservative conclusions.

As a result of the study, a few enhancements to the Visagraph system will be considered in the future, including the following:

- Employ a standard calibration routine to correct for detected issues with line assignments.
- Make adjustments to regressive incoming saccade and re-read definitions to align the system with current literature and gold-standard research devices.
- Increase the sample rate to capture smaller fixations.
- Implement an additional state-of-the-art digital presentation to help reduce inter-individual variation and to reflect today's task demands, as more and more reading is done from digital devices.

In conclusion, although there is some room for improvement in future development work, the study results indicate that the present Visagraph system produces practical and valid data within its intended area of reading performance analysis.

REFERENCES

Ahren, A. (1891). *Untersuchungen uber die bewegung der augen beim schreiben*, Rostock.

Aiken, C. (1896). *Methods of mind training.* New York: Harper and Brothers.

Anderson, I. H., & Dearborn, W. F. (1952). *The psychology of teaching reading.* New York: Ronald Press.

Ballantine, F. A. (1951). Age changes in measures of eye movements in silent reading. In *Studies of the psychology of reading.* (Monographs in Education, No. 4, pp. 67–111). Ann Arbor, MI: University of Michigan Press.

Barany, R. (1920). Apparat zur messung der rollbewegungen des auges. *Zeietschr F. Sinnesphsiol., 45,* 59.

Betts, E. A. (1946). *Foundations of reading instruction.* New York: American Book Company

Blythe, H. L., Liversedge, S. P., Joseph, H., White, S., Findlay, J. M., & Rayner, K. (2006). The binocular coordination of eye movements during reading in children and adults. *Vision Research, 46,* 3898–3909.

Brandt, H. F. (1945). *The psychology of seeing.* New York: The Philosophical Library.

Buswell, G. T. (1935). *How people look at pictures: A study of the psychology of perception in art.* Chicago: University of Chicago Press.

Buys, E. (1910–1911). Uber die nystagmographie beim menschen. *Internat. Zentralbl. F. Ohrenhk., 9,* pp. 57–65.

California State Department of Education. (1979). *Handbook for planning an effective reading program.* Sacramento, CA: Office of State Printing.

Carmichael, L., & Dearborn, W. F. (1947). *Reading and visual fatigue.* Boston: Houghton Mifflin.

Carver, R. P. (1989). Silent reading rates in grade equivalents. *Journal of Reading Behavior, XXI(2),* 155.

Cattell, J. (1885). The inertia of the eye and brain. *Brain, VIII,* 295–312.

Chomsky, C. (1976). After decoding: What? *Language Arts, 53*(3), 288–296, 314.

Ciuffreda, M. A., Ciuffreda, K. J., & Santos, D. (2003). Visagraph® baseline analysis and procedural guidelines. *Journal of Behavioral Optometry, 14*(3), 60–64.

Davis, L. F. (1956). The S.V.E. Speed-i-o-Scope, an investment for school learning. *Visual Review, 50*(1), *Society for Visual Education, 1*(7). *Journal of Educational Psychology, 94*(3), 474–485.

Dearborn, W. F. (1906). The psychology of reading, Columbia University *Contributions to Philosophy, Psychology and Education*, 14(1). Also listed in Archives of Philosophy. *Psychology and Scientific Methods, 4* (p. 134). New York: Columbia University Press.

Delabarre, E. B. (1898). A method of recording eye-movements. *American Journal of Psychology, 9*, 572–574.

Dodge, R. (1907). An experimental study of visual fixation. *Psychological Monograph, 8*, 1–95.

Dodge, R., & Cline, T. C. (1901, March). The angle velocity of eye-movements. *Psychological Review, 8*, 145–157.

Eide Neurolearning Blog. (September 9, 2012) http://eideneurolearningblog.blogspot.com/2009/09/visual-overload-and-visual-crowding.html.

Feinberg, R. (1949). A study of some aspects of peripheral visual acuity. *American Journal of Optometry and Archives of American Academy of Optometrics, 26*, 49–56.

Freeman, F. N. (1916). *Experimental education.* Boston: Houghton Mifflin.

Gates, A. I. (1935). *The improvement of reading.* New York: Macmillan.

George, E. J., Toren, J. A., & Lowell, J. W. (1923). Study of the ocular movements in the horizontal plane. *American Journal of Ophthalmology, 6*, 833–838.

Gilbert, D. W. (1956). *Power and Speed in Reading.* Englewood Cliffs, NJ: Prentice-Hall.

Gilbert, L. C. (1940, April). Effect on silent reading of attempting to follow oral reading. *Elementary School Journal, 40*, 614–621.

Gilbert, L. C. (1959a, February). Saccadic movements as a factor in visual perception in reading. *Journal of Educational Psychology, 50*, 15–19.

Gilbert, L. C. (1959b, February). Speed of processing visual stimuli and its relation to reading. *Journal of Educational Psychology, 50*, 8–14.

Gilbert, L. C., & Gilbert, D. W. (1942). Reading before the eye-movement camera versus reading away from it. *Elementary School Journal, 42*, 443–447.

Gray, C. T. (1917). Types of reading ability as exhibited through tests and laboratory experiments. *Supplementary Educational Monograph No. 5*, University of Chicago Press.

Gray, W. S. (1956). *The teaching of reading and writing* (pp. 53–59). Chicago: Scott, Foresman.

Grayum, H. S. (1953). What is skimming? What are its uses at different grade levels? *The Reading Teacher, 7*, 111–114.

Gross, E. G., Vaughan, Jr., H. G., & Valenstein, E. (1967). Inhibition of visual evoked responses to patterned stimuli during voluntary eye movements. *Electroence phalography and Clinical Neurophysiology, 22*(3), 204–209.

Guilford, J. B., & Hackman, R. B. (1936, July). Varieties and levels of clearness correlated with eye movements. *American Journal of Psychology, 48*, 371–388.

Heller, D., & Radach, R. (1999). Eye movements in reading: Are two eyes better than one? In W. Becker, H. Deubel, & T. Mergner (Eds.), *Current oculomotor research: Physiological and psychological aspects* (pp. 341–348). New York: Plenum Press.

Hellerstein, L. F., Danner, R., Maples, W. C., Press, L., Schneebeck, J., & Miller, S. (2001, Summer). Optometric guidelines for school consulting. *Journal of Optometric Vision Development, 32*(2), 56–75.

Hoffman, A. C., Wellman, B., & Carmichael, L. (1939). A quantitative comparison of the electrical and photographic techniques of eye-movement recording. *Journal of Experimental Psychology, 24*, 40–53.

Hoffman, J. E., & Subramaniam, B. (1995). The role of visual attention in saccadic eye movements. *Perception & Psychophysics, 57*, 787–795.

Holland, B. F. (1927, October). Special apparatus in the laboratory of educational psychology, University of Texas. *American Journal of Psychology, 27*, 534–583.

Hoover, C. D., & Harris, P. (1997, Winter). The effects of using the ReadFast computer program on eye movement abilities as measured by the OBER2 eye movement device. *Journal of Optometric Vision Development, 28*, 227–234.

Huestegge, L., Radach, R., Corbie, D., & Huestegge, S. M. (2009). Oculomotor and linguistic determinants of reading development: A longitudinal study. *Vision Research, 40*, 2948–4959.

Huey, E. B. (1898). Preliminary experiments in the physiology and psychology of reading. *American Journal of Psychology, 9*, 575–586.j

Huey, E. B. (1908). *The psychology and pedagogy of reading.* New York: Macmillan. Republished by the MIT Press, Cambridge, MA.

James, W. (1890). *The principles of psychology*, Vol.1. New York: Henry Holt.

Javal, L. E. (1879). Essai sur la Physiologie de la lecture. *Annales d'Oculistique, 82*, 242–253.

Judd, C. H., McAllister, C. N., & Steele, W. M. (1905). General introduction to a series of studies of eye-movements by means of kinetoscopic photographs. *Phycological Monograph, 7*, 1–16.

Kliegl, R., Nuthmann, A., & Engbert, R. (2006). Tracking the mind during reading: The influence of past, present, and future words on fixation durations. *Journal of Experimental Psychology: General, 135*, 12–35.

LaBerge, D., & Samuels, S. J. (1974). Toward a theory of automatic information processing in reading. *Cognitive Psychology, 6*(2), 293–323.

Lamare, A. (1892). Des movements des yeux dans la lecture. *Bull. Mem. Soc. Franc. d'Ophtal., 10*, 354–364.

Learner, K. M., & Richman, C. L. (1984). The effect of modifying the cognitive tempo of reading disabled children on reading comprehension. *Contemporary Educational Psychology, 9*(2), 122–134.

Legge, G. E., Cheung, S.-H., Yu, D., Chung, S. T. L., Lee, H.-W., & Owens, D. P. (2007). The case for the visual span as a sensory bottleneck in reading. *Journal of Vision, 7*(2):9, 1–15.

Litterer, O. F. (1932). An experimental analysis of reading performance. *Journal of Experimental Education, 1*, 28–37.

Logan, G. O. (1997). Automaticity and reading: Perspectives from the instance theory of automaticity. *Reading and Writing Quarterly, 13*, 123–146.

Maples, W. C., & Hoenes, R. (2009). The College of Optometrists in Vision Development checklist related to vision function: Expert opinions. *Optometry, 80*(12): 688–694.

McConkie, G. W., & Rayner, K. (1976). Asymmetry of the perceptual span in reading. *Bulletin of the Psychometric Society, 8,* 365–368.

McConkie, G. W., & Zola, D. (1989). Some characteristics of readers' eye movements. In C. von Euler, I. Lundberg, & G. Lennerstrand (Eds.), *Brain and reading* (pp. 369–381). London: Macmillan.

Miles, W. R. (1928). The peep-hole method of observing eye-movements in reading. *Journal of General Psychology, 1,* 373–374.

Miles, W. R., & Shen, E. (1925). Photographic recording of eye movements in the reading of Chinese in vertical and horizontal axes: Method and preliminary results. *Journal and Experimental Psychology, 8,* 344–362.

Miller, G. A. (1956). The magic number seven, plus or minus two: Some limits on our capacity for processing information. *Psychological Review, 63,* 81–97.

Morris, H. F. (1973). *Eye-movement analysis with the Reading Eye II.* New York: EDL/McGraw-Hill.

Morse, W. C. (1951). Comparisons of the eye movements of fifth and seventh grade pupils reading materials of corresponding difficulty. In *Studies in the Psychology of Reading. Monographs in Education, No. 4* (pp. 3–64). Ann Arbor, MI: University of Michigan Press.

National Home Education Research Institute. (September 10, 2012). http://www.nheri.org/research/research-facts-on-homeschooling.html.

National Institute of Child Health and Human Development. (2000). *Report of the National Reading Panel. Teaching children to read: An evidence-based assessment of the scientific research literature on reading and its implications for reading instruction: Report of the subgroups* (NIH Publication No. 00–4769). Washington, DC: U. S. Government Printing Office.

National Parent Teacher Association. (1999, June). Learning related vision problems education and evaluation resolution adopted at the Network PTA Convention.

Norman D. A., & Bobrow, D. G. (1975). On data-limited and resource-limited processes. *Cognitive Psychology 7,* 44–64.

Ohm, J. (1914). Zur graphischen registrierung des augen zitterns der bergleute und der lidbewegungen, *Zeitschr. F. Augenheilk, 32,* 4–8.

Pavlidis, G. T., & Miles, T. R. (1981). *Dyslexia research and its applications to education.* New York: John Wiley & Sons.

Posner, M. I. (1980). Orienting of attention. *Quarterly Journal of Experimental Psychology, 32,* 3–25.

Radach, R., Reilly, R., & Inhoff, A. W. (2007). Models of oculomotor control in reading: Towards a theoretical foundation of current debates. In R. van Gompel, M. Fischer, W. Murray, & R. Hill (Eds.), *Eye movements: A window on mind and brain* (pp. 237–270). Oxford, England: Elsevier.

Rayner, K. (1983). Eye movements, perceptual span, and reading disability. *Annals of Dyslexia, 33,* 163–73.

Rayner, K., & Morrison, R. (1981). Eye movements and identifying words in parafoveal vision. *Bulletin of the Psychonomic Society, 17,* 135–138.

Rayner, K., Pollatsek, A., Ashby, J., & Clifton, C. (2012). *Psychology of reading* Psychology Press.

Rusk, R. R. (1915). A Tachistoscope for class experiment and demonstration purposes. *Journal of Educational Psychology, VI,* 429–431.

Samuels, S. J. (2006). Toward a model of reading fluency. In S. J. Samuels & A. E. Farstrup (Eds.), *What research has to say about fluency instruction* (pp. 24–46). Newark, DE: International Reading Association.

Schlange, D., Patel, H., & Caden, B. (1999). Evaluation of the Reading Plus 2000 and Visagraph System as a remedial program for academically "at risk" sixth and eighth grade students: A pilot study. *Optometry and Vision Science, 76,* poster 11.

Seibert, E. W. (1943). Reading reactions for varied types of subject matter. *Journal of Experimental Education, 12,* 37–44.

Shelley-Tremblay, J., & Eyer, J. (2009). Effect of the Reading Plus program on reading skills in second graders. *Journal of Behavioral Optometry, 20*(3), 59–66.

Solan, H. A., Hansen, P., Shelley-Tremblay, J., & Ficarra, A. (2004). M-cell deficit and reading disability: A preliminary study of the effects of temporal vision-processing therapy. *Optometry, 75,* 640–650.

Storm, G. E., & Smith, N. B. (1930). *Reading activities in the primary grades.* Boston: Ginn.

Tannen, B. M., & Ciuffreda, K. J. (2007). A proposed addition to the standard protocol for the Visagraph® II eye movement recording system. *Journal of Behavioral Optometry, 18(6),* 143–147.

Taylor, E. A. (1937). *Controlled reading.* Chicago: University of Chicago Press.

Taylor, E. A. (1966). *The fundamental reading skill* (2nd ed.), xviii, 157. Springfield, IL: Charles C Thomas.

Taylor E. A., & Solan, H. A. (1956). *Functional readiness and school adjustment.* New York: Reading and Study Skills Center.

Taylor, S. E. (1960). *Eye-movement photography with the Reading Eye.* Huntington, NY: Educational Development Laboratories, Inc.

Taylor, S. E. (1962, May). Reading instrument usage. *The Reading Teacher,* 15, 449–54.

Taylor, S. E. (1976–1978). National study of fluency in the primary grades. Instructional Communications Technology Research and Information Brief.

Taylor, S. E. (1981). National study of fluency in the primary grades, Phase II Final Report–School Year 1978–1981, *I/CT Teacher Education Monograph No. 11.* Huntington Station, NY: Instructional/Communications Technology, Inc.

Taylor, S. E. (2011). *Exploring silent reading fluency: Its nature and development.* Springfield, IL: Charles C Thomas.

Taylor, S. E., Frackenpohl, H., & Pettee, J. L. (1959). A report on two studies of the validity of eye-movement photography as a measurement of reading performance. *Reading in a Changing Society, International Reading Association Conference Proceeding, 4.*

Taylor, S. E., Frackenpohl, H., & Pettee, J. L. (1960). Grade level norms for the components of the fundamental reading skills. *EDL Research and Information Bulletin, No. 3,* 22. New York: EDL/McGraw-Hill.

Taylor, S. E., & Robinson, H. A. (1963, February). The relationship of the oculomotor efficiency of the beginning reader to his success in learning to read. Paper presented at the meeting of the American Educational Research Association, Chicago, IL.

Tinker, M. A. (1931). Apparatus for recording eye movements. *American Journal of Psychology, 43*, 115–118.

Travis, R. C. (1932, October). Experimental studies in ocular behavior, I: The Dodge Mirror-Recorder for photographing eye-movements. *Journal of General Psychology, 7*, 311–327.

Vernon, M. D. (1930, July). An apparatus for the photographic recording of eye-movements. *British Journal of Psychology, 21*, 65.

Volkmann, A. W. (1859). Das Tachistoskop, ein Instrument, Welches bei Untersuchung des Momentanen Sehens den Gebrauch de Elektrischens Funkens Ersetzt. Berichte Uber die Verhandlungen der Koniglich Sachischen Gesellschaft der Wissenschaften Zu Leipzig (Math. Phys. Classe) 90–98 (As given by Cassie Spencer Payne).

Volkmann, F. C. (1962). Vision during voluntary saccadic eye movements. *Optical Society of America Journal, 52*(5), 571–578.

Weber, C. O. (1937). The use of tachistoscopic exercise in the improvement of reading. *Psychological Bulletin, XXXIV*, 533–534.

West, R. F. (1978). *Efficient processing activities in reading.* Newark, DE: The International Reading Association.

Wilkins, M. C. (1917). A tachistoscopic experiment in reading. Unpublished master's thesis, Columbia University, 24.

Yarbus, A. L. (1967). *Eye movements and vision.* New York: Plenum Press.

INDEX

H

I

J

K

L

M

N

O

P

R

S